Inside Our

Broken Healthcare System

By: Linda M. Girgis, MD, FAAFP

book cover artist: SelfPubBookCovers.com/Phantom

For those who inspired me;

For those who gave me my voice;

For those who didn't quit on me....or let me quit;

For those on the frontlines of medicine, fighting

this fight every day;

For patients everywhere, you deserve better.

There are simply no words that can be said to express my

gratitude!

Table of Contents

Disclaimer: Medical facts on patients have been slightly altered to protect HIPAA rights.

Preface

Inside the Broken Healthcare System

Inside Our Broken Healthcare System

After spending a week of fighting and making multiple phone calls, I feel a certain victory in finally getting approval for a MRI I know my patient needs to accurately diagnose her symptoms. Until I realize that a week has been lost in initiating treatment and relieving this patient's pain because of the red tape that now ensues after ordering specific diagnostic tests. And another stack of medication prior authorizations wait for my review. The one in front of me is for an asthma medication. The insurance company is requesting that I change to a medication that does not even have the same mechanism of action. From my experience, I know my efforts at getting this medication covered will be denied. And my patient will be unable to afford the exorbitant out-of-pocket costs. What typically happens is that the patient has to first fail on the alternative drug. What is a drug failure in the insurance company's eyes is more like weeks of cough, wheezing, and not being able to breath in my patient's. Gone are the days when doctors are able to do the best for our patients. Medical decision-making on many levels has been torn from our authority, to be replaced by case managers and insurance company employees whose main goal is to keep costs down.

Few people would argue that the American healthcare system is in need of repairs. Our country has some of the highest medical advances and technology in the world. Yet, patients are not always utilizing these cutting edge treatments because inefficiencies in our healthcare system are preventing them from doing so. Patients are increasingly disgruntled at having services for diagnostic tests and coverage for their prescription medications denied. In some areas, it is even difficult for them to find access to doctors they need.

Doctors are similarly disenchanted with their chosen careers. After long years of study and huge amounts of debt, they are finding that they are not able to practice medicine the way they truly feel is the best for their patients. Additionally, burnout rates among physicians are high as regulatory burdens rise, insurance companies make getting paid more difficult and reimbursements stagnate or decrease. Meanwhile, overhead costs continue to soar.

How did the best healthcare system decay to such a chaotic state?

Inside Our Broken Healthcare System

Many say it is the fault of doctors who do procedures for profit and are driven to make more money. Even our Commander-in-Chief, President Obama, made this accusation in one of his Presidential speeches. Yet, only 20% of healthcare dollars go to physicians and half of this 20% goes to covering overhead expenses. Contrary to some peoples' belief, most doctors truly have the patients' best interests at heart. We work many hours, much of it uncompensated. When your doctor sends your refills without making you come for an office visit or answers your urgent calls at 3 am, we get paid nothing for that. We do it because it is to offer patients the best care. We are often on call over-night and holidays, many times for no additional pay. Sure, there are some outlier doctors who game the system. But, in my experience, this is a very small number.

Perhaps, the biggest damage to the healthcare system came with the arrival of HMOs. These are organizations that are designed to control costs, often by denying expensive care and medications. Keeping costs down is very important. However, there are some patients who need these procedures and medications. Yet, much is spent on employing people for managing doctors' decisions so we don't bankrupt the system. Meanwhile, the insurance company executives earn millions from this denied care and they are accountable to no one. While there is oversight on physicians' practicing habits, there is none of how insurance companies profit. Perhaps, true healthcare reform should bring these companies under tighter scrutiny?

Another harmful effect on the medical system is the Big Brother regulations set in place by the government. Most people have heard the woes of Medicare and there are always predictions on when it will go bankrupt. It consumes much healthcare dollars without adding much quality to healthcare. Rather, these funds are put into increasing bureaucracy and red tape, for doctors and patients alike. For example, there is now a push to have EHRs in every medical practice. New guidelines have been published and criteria set that needs to be met. Unfortunately, many of the software systems simply cannot perform the functions the government is requiring for such things as their meaningful use

program. Much money is being spent on refining and revising this,

yet doctors all across the nation are crying out that their guidelines

are not helpful and meaningful. And to input them into the patient

chart, it takes time away from direct patient care. Is it better we

spend time face to face with our patients listening to their

concerns, or check marking the boxes in the chart that the

government wants us to meet their requirements?

These are just a few examples of what we have seen already but

soon we are going to have a true crisis of access to care. More

doctors are getting frustrated and retiring early or quitting

medicine. The ACA has enrolled more insured patients. But, more

doctors are not being trained. Who is going to take care of all these

patients? Many patients turn to the ER when they can't get in with

their private doctor. ERs are already over-burdened. Surely

something must give before this leads to a true disaster.

While many things are broken in the healthcare system and many

doctors dread going to work, patients are the biggest losers here.

They are no longer seen as people but as consumers and people seem more concerned about their data. Doctors have made some attempts to change the system but have often failed to the big corporations. Maybe, the only way change will come if patients do likewise and demand the level of care they deserve.

And as the pile of paperwork is completed, I head to the exam room to see the next patient. I remind myself why I became a doctor: for that patient waiting for me in the exam room. That patient will never be a consumer or a set of data to me but rather a person who entrusted me to help make the best medical decisions for them. And I will continue to fight the broken system every day, no matter what it takes, because patients deserve better than what they are receiving.

Chapter 1: The Problem of the

Uninsured

Inside Our Broken Healthcare System

The patient was having severe abdominal pain. Clearly, this was not something that could be managed in an out-patient setting. However, the patient was refusing to go to the emergency room because they did not have any insurance. After a prolonged discussion of the risks including the possibility of appendicitis, he reluctantly agreed.

What happens when the uninsured patient goes to the ER? They will be treated the same as someone who has insurance. Sometimes, if the patient is below a certain income level, they can be placed on charity care and not have to pay anything. The hospital receives certain funds to cover these patients. The larger proportion, however, will not qualify. And many of them just simply cannot afford to pay their hospital bills. Oftentimes, these medical expenses simply go unpaid and the hospital ends up writing off the costs.

But, it does not stop there. Hospitals cannot afford to keep eating these huge costs. They have high overhead expenses to pay and employees who need to collect their salaries and benefits. The costs get spread to the payers, whether the patient or covering insurance company. The cost of providing medical care to those with no health care coverage has indeed been shown to drive up the costs for the entire healthcare system. It has been estimated that 55% of ER costs now go uncompensated. This is because the ER serves as a safety- net. It is a legal requirement that they must treat all patients regardless of their insurance status or their ability to pay. As we all know, the ACA (Affordable Care Act), also known as ObamaCare, went into effect in early 2014. The ACA was postulated to ameliorate the problem of the uninsured. Everyone is now required to have health insurance, whether through their workplaces or privately purchased, or face tax penalties. The tax penalties start out small but grow year by year. Despite this new law, many people are still choosing to go bare. Many people simply cannot afford the cost of the premium and wish to try their luck with the tax penalties. They are struggling to pay their already existent expenses and just do not have any more money. Others are refusing to sign up for coverage based on principle: they disagree with the ACA. The problem is basically shifted back unto the people to correct. The first enrollment period occurred early in 2014 and was wrought with chaos. People were on hold for hours trying to get information to enroll, the website had technological glitches, and people just had a downright impossible task getting accurate data. Obviously, the problem of the uninsured is not going away any time soon.

Another problem I have seen with patients who don't have insurance is the inability to get in to see specialists. Recently, I had a patient with a neurological problem who I felt needed to see a neurologist quickly. When calling around to refer the patient, no one wanted to see the patient because they lacked health insurance coverage. This was a patient willing to pay out of pocket. But, many of the specialists' offices were just not listening to that. Surely, they have been burned with outstanding balances in the past. But, this patient needed urgent care, not necessarily emergency room care. Yet, that is where this patient indeed ended up going.

Why is the number of uninsured patients an indication of a broken healthcare system?

- As stated above, these patients often seek medical care in the ER and not in a traditional office setting. They simply cannot find a doctor to see them or one that will see them for free. There is a definite lack of access for them into traditional medical settings.

- Many of them will end up defaulting on their ER bills. This is a major financial loss for the treating hospital. ERs are already overwhelmed in the number of patients they are treating and they should be reserved for true emergencies. Hospitals have been struggling to stay afloat and write offs impact an already stressed hospital's economics. It is also impacts the economics of the healthcare system as a whole.

- The uninsured create a true disparity in health care. Many of them cannot afford the diagnostic tests that are recommended for their symptoms. By virtue of their lack of insurance, they are often offered less medical services based on their ability to pay. Diseases do not discriminate on socio-economic basis. Treatment and diagnostic services should be the same across the board. But, this is simply not possible when patients cannot foot the bill.

- There are some who feel that healthcare is a basic human right that everyone is entitled to have. This is not possible in our present broken system. Some will have coverage, some will not.

- Our current system tends to exclude those who have less money. It has been hotly debated whether healthcare is a right or not. But, as it stands currently, those with less money are left out of many medical services.

While the problem of the uninsured is a real, valid concern, no good solution exists. While the ACA had the eradication of the uninsured as one of its goals, it obviously did not succeed in achieving this objective. Novel ways need to be explored to address how this problem is adversely affecting our already broken system. Patients need to step up and take some responsibility for their own health but efforts also need to be made to make it more affordable. People should have access to quality healthcare, but they should not expect it for free. It is time that both sides find a compromising answer to the problem of the uninsured.

There is an additional problem in that some of the uninsured are undocumented immigrants. I have seen several coming to me with serious conditions because they were afraid to go to the ER because of their immigration status. These patients have limited resources. Many of them are struggling with language and cultural barriers. Many of them do not understand the nuances of the American healthcare system. For this reason, many avoid medical care until a true crisis situation develops. And then they end up in the ER, which further drives up the cost of care.

I have seen several women come with huge breast masses because they put off their medical care because they felt they could not afford it. What was in essence probably a curable disease if they came when they first noted a problem, now becomes a terminal illness. The prognosis is much worse, the treatment much more complicated, and, again, this drives up healthcare costs.

Inside Our Broken Healthcare System

According to a Gallup poll, the second quarter of 2014 saw a drop in the uninsured rate to 13.4%. While the number of uninsured is reduced, more than 10% of the US population still has no medical insurance coverage. This is a very significant number and represents a huge burden on the healthcare system. This number does not reflect the disparity across different demographic groups. For example, 33.2% of Hispanics remain uninsured, the largest demographic group to lack insurance. In lower income households, defined as having annual incomes less than $36,000, 25.2% remained uninsured. Not only does this show the significant number of uninsured, but it displays the true disparities among those covered. 1

According to government estimates, there are nearly 46 million uninsured people in the US, 20% (8.7 million) are children. Many of these are in households where the parents work but just cannot afford to purchase insurance and do not qualify for public programs. CMS predicts that the cost of the uninsured will reach $176 billion dollars by the end of 2014. Given these statistics, it is very easy to see the huge scope of this problem and the impact that it is playing on the healthcare system. 2

In addition to people not being able to afford a new premium payment, employers are having a difficult time subsidizing insurance payments. They are putting more of the costs back on their employees. Health insurance premiums are especially impacting small businesses and many of them just cannot afford to offer it to their employees any longer. Many workers now seek health care benefits when seeking employment, rather than the amount of their wages. It is getting more difficult for small businesses to compete and stay in business.

It is not only the uninsured patients who are having a difficult time paying their medical bills but insured people are as well. Many plans now have large deductibles. Also, many services are no longer paid by insurance companies. This is especially true for patients with rare or uncommon diseases. Many of the treatments for these diseases are considered experimental and thus exempted from insurance coverage. And often these treatments are very expensive and the only hope many of these patients have. Many go into debt trying to get well or taking care of a sick family member. In fact, it is estimated that 1.5 million people will file bankruptcy in 2014 because of medical bills. Truly, someone should not lose all they have in a quest for a cure. There needs to be help here. For years, patients have become accustomed to paying only a co-pay. Under the health insurance exchanges, patients are bearing the burden of higher costs. More patients are now paying a significant portion of their insurance premiums. At the same time, many of these plans have much higher deductibles and patients are paying more out-of-pocket expenses. I have seen many irate patients in my practice who just didn't realize that they were responsible for paying for these costs. Most people understand the new rules, but those who don't are truly disillusioned. This is proving to be very significant hurdle for many patients. Sometimes, they need to decide whether the medical treatment they are seeking is truly worth spending the money to obtain. Their medical well-being becomes a budgeted item rather than a right.

Inside Our Broken Healthcare System

I recently saw a woman who was scheduled for follow up of her high blood pressure. It was an important visit for her to keep because we were adjusting her medication to try to better control her blood pressure. She cancelled this visit and told my receptionist that her child was sick and she needed to take him to his pediatrician. She was unable to afford the deductibles for both visits.

Likewise, I saw another woman who was having abdominal pain for several weeks. She was diagnosed with gallbladder disease and told that she needed surgery to remove her gall bladder. However, when evaluating her out-of-pocket expenses, she determined that she was simply unable to afford it. Rather, she continues with her abdominal pain and other symptoms. In her case, she will live with the pain or end up in the ER when a complication sets in. Neither of these options is acceptable in my opinion.

How can patients' expectations be brought to reality?

- When a person signs an insurance contract, they should understand the exact terms of what they are signing. This holds true for anything, not just insurance contracts. If someone is unaware that they have a deductible, it will not make it go away. They are liable to pay all deductibles and it would behoove everyone if both sides try to make sure this is clear.

- Doctors need to inform the patient up front that they have a deductible. We do this prior to seeing the patient so they are aware that they will be responsible for paying a certain amount.

– Medical office staff needs to understand these rules and be able to explain them to patients. It is not enough just to tell the patient they owe a certain amount of money. The staff needs to be able to explain why.

Inside Our Broken Healthcare System

- Insurance cards should have the deductible written on them along with the copay. Most patients pull out their cards and say that according to this, they are just responsible for the copay. This is in fact not always true. The benefits and responsibilities should be clearly written on the card so there is no confusion.

-Insurance companies should have support staff available to answer patient questions about coverage. We hear all too often that the patient did try to call their insurance company and were unable to speak to a live person. They were placed on hold for unreasonable amounts of time and then not given accurate information.

The new insurance exchanges that have been rolled out have been fraught with many problems that we are all aware from media outlets. However, we are now starting to see some of the impact it is playing in our daily lives. Patients are unhappy because they are responsible for subsidizing a larger part of their healthcare costs. And for many of them, their expectations were not set at an appropriate level to start with. This has led to some bitter exchanges with the office staff, who are not happy for this reason

Additionally, physicians are not happy because all too often this means getting paid in a less than timely fashion, if at all, for work that we are fully entitled to receive payment. The new deductibles are indeed placing a burden on many and something needs to be done before more chaos ensues. The middle class is being especially squeezed.

As discussed, the problem of the uninsured is both a symptom of the broken healthcare system while at the same time being one of its biggest contributors. The ACA has failed to fix this problem and clearly a better solution is needed. Until this repair happens, hospitals will continue losing money and patients will keep seeking care at more advanced stages of illness. These both will continue to drive up healthcare costs. It has also been shown that those who lack health insurance coverage do not get preventive or screening procedures done. If things continue as they are, surely a breaking point will come when hospitals can no longer afford to do business this way. By law, they cannot deny medical services to anyone, regardless of their ability to pay. An answer is urgently needed.

This problem, like we have discussed, is not only with the uninsured but with the under-insured as well. Patients are putting off treatments and procedures because of their lack of funds. This too will drive up healthcare costs as they present with diseases at more advanced stages and with more complications. Unlike ERs, medical practices and doctors are not required to treat those that cannot afford to pay. Clearly, the health insurance industry is an instigator in this problem as we shall explore further in the following chapters.

1-http://www.gallup.com/poll/168821/uninsured-rate-drops.aspx

2- http://www.acep.org/News-Media-top-banner/The-Uninsured-
-Access-To-Medical-Care/

Chapter 2: For Profit Insurance

Companies

Inside Our Broken Healthcare System

Many patients assume that doctors make tons of money. While we are well off for the most part, we are not among the richest. We cannot afford yachts and weekly golf outings. We do not all drive Lamborghinis. The truth is that physicians' salaries have stayed the same or decreased over the past decade. Yet, inflation and the cost of living have soared. And there are many doctors financially strapped, especially those trying to keep their private practices afloat. Overhead costs have been soaring as have employee salaries.

People look at the cost of their insurance premiums and cast blame on doctors for these high costs. Yet, much of their premium dollars do not go to the physicians. The latest statistics available from CMS is from 2013. Total healthcare spending increased 3.6% from the previous year, reaching a total of $2.9 trillion, which is equivalent to $9,255 per person. Hospital spending increased to $936.9 billion while the spending on doctors and clinical services increased to $586.7 billion. Prescription drugs cost another $271.1 billion and durable medical equipment $43 billion in the same time period. The complete statistical picture can be seen on the CMS

website. 1 It is clear from these statistics that there are healthcare

dollars going to many places and doctors represent just a small

piece of this.

How big are health insurance company profits?

According to an article in the NYT in November 2014, the answer

is huge. United Healthcare (UHC), Medicaid, and Medicare

Advantage are expected to generate $60 BILLION in revenue by the

end of 2014. UHC has added over 1 million new members to its

Medicaid plans and expects to expand its health insurance

exchange coverage to 23 states next year, up from 4 in 2014.

Wellpoint gained 751,000 new subscribers under the health

insurance exchanges and 699,000 new members through Medicaid.

2   Aetna has similarly shown a rise in profits under the ACA, and its

profits rose to $58.8 million in the previous quarter. 3

Inside Our Broken Healthcare System

And it not just the insurance companies that are raking in the huge profits but their top executives are as well. The biggest winner appears to be Aetna's CEO, Mark Bertolini, who earned $30.7 MILLION in 2013, up from the previous year's salary of $13.3 million, representing a 131% raise. The CEO's of Wellpoint, Cigna, Centene, UHC and Molina all received salaries over $10 million for 2013, while others followed at only $7 or $8 million. The average salary of health insurance CEO's in 2013 was $13,886.71 Million. 4

I doubt that anyone would fail to see the financial conflict of interest here. When the CEO earns over $30 MILLION, one has to wonder if some of this money could be better used saving lives. The next time your doctor orders a CT scan of your belly because you have pain and it is denied, you have to wonder how many CT scans could be done with those millions of dollars those executives are raking in.

Inherit in the concept of private insurance companies is the idea to reduce healthcare costs and maximize profits. There is a financial incentive for insurance companies to deny care (this will be discussed further in the next chapter). I think few would argue that

insurance companies function as corporations and are looking at

maximizing their bottom line. But this is where an ethical dilemma

sets in. An insurance company is unique from other corporations

because their decisions can affect the life and health of real

patients. Patients can die when wrong decisions are made. Yet,

insurance companies continue to make these decisions, without

actually taking a medical history or physical exam, on a daily basis.

And their decisions and guidelines are driven by costs and profits. I

think few would fail to see the wrong in this. Big corporations

should not be optimizing profits by making medical decisions that

can harm patients. In the same vein, making all these guidelines

and enforcing them is driving up costs as well. How many

employees does an insurance company have that is responsible for

prior authorizations and its related tasks? How much is this costing

the system? I would be very interested to know, for instance, the

cost of a MRI as compared to the costs of a denial of one. I imagine

the costs of the paperwork burden a substantial one. And, often, these decisions are not decided by doctors but rather non-medically trained employees of health insurance companies.

And despite the fact that the ACA was purported to save healthcare costs, commercial insurers were the ones who gained the most from its passage.

Why commercial insurance plans are the biggest winners under the ACA?

- They are collecting unprecedented number of premiums. Many people are paying these premiums even though they do not want to. They feel coerced into it because they wish to avoid a tax penalty. There is no government oversight to how much these health insurances can charge. While now the market is very competitive, I expect costs to rise as the market gets saturated.

– They are paying out less for medical services. Virtually all the plans I have seen, require the patient to pay a high deductible before they pay for any services. Many patients are forgoing care just because they cannot afford both their new premiums and the deductibles. In many cases these deductibles are quite high and the chances that the insurance company will pay out anything will be minimal.

– Medicaid is increasingly enrolling those eligible through HMO's via the insurance exchanges. Not only are these exchanges getting private dollars, they are now collecting state money. Where I practice, there are very few patients who have only Medicaid not issued through a HMO.

– Private insurance is for profit. They can collect as much money as they want. They are incentivized to collect more and pay out less. The more money they make, the more money they can keep for themselves.

– Unlike Medicare and Medicaid, there is little oversight over these private insurance companies.

While many proclaim the goodness of the ACA getting insurance for the uninsured, it is not without its faults. Sure, more people are insured but they are being insured by paying more money out of their own pockets. Many of them are struggling to make these premiums and are further frustrated by the fact they are unable to see the doctor due to high deductibles. So, despite having insurance, many simply can still not afford to come for medical care. The people the ACA is supposed to be helping, the patient, are being more squeezed by it in many way.

The **PCP** (primary care physician) as the gatekeeper, as it was previously known, or the **PCMH** (patient centered medical home) as it is now known is another interesting area to contemplate. Under these plans, a patient must first see a PCP and get a referral to see any specialist. While this is good in some regards, it should not be so stringent across the board. I recently saw a young boy who fractured his arm. He was seen in the ER and told to see the orthopedist. But, in order to see the orthopedist, he has to come to see me first to do the referral. And because I have never seen him before, he had to have an office visit. This is a situation where it makes more sense, both medically and financially, for the patient to see the orthopedist based on the recommendation of the doctor in the ER.

Huge profits earned by over-riding doctors' medical decisions are also a symptom of the broken system and a big contributor to the damage. While they will deny it, insurance companies are basically practicing medicine when they choose to make a decision about whether or not a patient needs a certain diagnostic test or procedure performed. They will tell you that they are only determining coverage, not making medical decisions. But, let's face facts. If a patient could afford these tests out-of-pocket, there would be no need for health insurance coverage. And the vast majority of patients simply will not do it if the insurance company does not cover it. Perhaps, the time is here to expand the role of non-profit health insurance companies in the US healthcare marketplace. Additionally, the salaries of health insurance companies should become more transparent and be more scrutinized. True healthcare reform will occur only when insurance companies are reformed and subject to regulatory over-sight.

1- . http://www.cms.gov/Research-Statistics-Data-and-Systems/Statistics-Trends-and-Reports/NationalHealthExpendData/downloads/highlights.pdf
2- http://www.nytimes.com/2014/11/18/us/politics/health-law-turns-obama-and-insurers-into-allies.html
3- http://www.nytimes.com/2014/11/18/us/politics/health-law-turns-obama-and-insurers-into-allies.html

4- . http://www.healthcare-now.org/health-insurance-ceo-pay-skyrockets-in-2013

Chapter 3: Denied Care

Inside Our Broken Healthcare System

Imagine that you have been suffering for weeks to months with headaches, abdominal pain, or some other such symptom which is making your life miserable. Now, you are starting to get worried about it because you don't know what it causing it. Perhaps, it is not just a migraine again but maybe something more dire, like cancer. You make the appointment and go see your doctor who explains what needs to be done next and your options. You and your doctor decide on a course of action that you both agree upon. Your doctor is also concerned and advises you to have a certain test done to diagnose your problem. But what happens next?

It would be simple if the test got scheduled in a relatively quick manner so you can stop losing sleep over not knowing what is wrong with you. First, however, you medical insurance company needs to approve that test. And many times, it gets flat-out denied without any review of the chart or the notes as medically unnecessary. And, by someone who is not even a doctor and never saw you, the patient. The decision that you and your doctor agreed upon is completely cast aside. Many times it takes the insurance 2-3 days to give you that denial.

There are times when a doctor can get on the phone with the medical director of that insurance company. It happened to me today as it has many days in the recent past. A woman was suffering from pain and I felt it was urgent that she get a STAT CT scan done. After a lengthy battle with the medical director, it was denied. I pointed out all the reasons she needed it done and it may be harmful to her health to delay the diagnosis. However, the patient did not fit in with the insurance company's treatment pathway to allow for such a test, a pathway designed to keep costs down, not improve the health of its insured members.

What can be done next? The patient can have a less expensive test, which probably will not reveal if there is really a problem. Or she can go to the ER where her costs will probably be 10 times what the requested test would have cost. Unless, the patient rather choose to just continue to suffer.

Inside Our Broken Healthcare System

Denials of tests and procedures are happening at an increasingly alarming rate. Sure it is important to try to keep healthcare costs contained and avoid unnecessary tests, but not at the expense of quality care for the patients. If anyone wants to look at the salaries of the executives of these insurance companies, it will give a good impression of what is driving these denials in these big for profit companies.

In the US, we have some of the best advances in medicine across the globe. But what good is it if patients are continually denied access to them? As a doctor, I try to do the best for my patients. It is getting increasingly more difficult when my hands are so often tied by the companies that are supposed to be saving lives. While these battles wear me down, I will continue to wage them because my patients deserve quality medical care. Perhaps the time has come for patients to demand more from this broken system. All patients deserve much more than what they are getting. Do we really want to let those whose main goals are to cut costs making our healthcare decisions for us?

A good example can be seen in the following case. "According to our company's guidelines, the patient needs to try 6 weeks of physical therapy first", said the medical director of a certain insurance company during a peer-to-peer phone conversation as they are called. And I truly did know that most cases of back pain should go to the physical therapist first before going to the MRI. But, the patient in front of me, for who I was fighting coverage for a test I thought necessary, did not look like he fit on the company's clinical pathway. For one thing, he was in too much pain to actually stand up, yet alone get in a car to drive to the physical therapist. And, he had some unusual numbness in his leg that raised a red flag in my mind that this is indeed something more perilous than just a lumbar muscle strain. No matter how I pleaded the case, the medical director just wasn't budging on the decision. In my mind, I was wondering if he would have considered the case differently if he had actually examined and spoke with the patient, rather than just reviewing his data. In the end,   the MRI was denied and I had to be the one to face the patient and tell him the news. The patient ended up leaving the visit in pain and dissatisfied, not receiving the medical care that he wanted and needed. Later that day, the patient had a worsening of pain and ended up the ER, where an emergent MRI was done. So not only did the denial of this test put my patient at increased risk, it drove up the cost of his medical care. I can probably tell a similar story many times a week.

Lately, it seems that more and more tests are being denied. It used to be that when I spoke with the medical director personally and explained the patient's history, the test would be authorized. This is not happening so often anymore. It becomes a battle on the phone. I feel all too often I am waging war on behalf of my patients with someone who never evaluated the patient. Yet, the doctor on the other end of the telephone bears no responsibility in the outcome. He is pretty much protected from liability by the insurance contracts. And, it is all too frequently told to me, if the test is necessary, the patient can pay out of pocket. The insurance company is only determining coverage and not making medical decisions. However, most patients simply cannot afford many of these tests. What is the point of having insurance if needed

treatments are going to be arbitrarily denied? But, it indeed gets

the medical director and insurance company off the hook if

something goes wrong.

And it is not just diagnostic tests being denied. I have a woman who

was told that she needs a hip replacement. She had an x-ray that

shows she has severe degenerative arthritis of her hip. She is

constantly in severe pain and this has limited her ability to work.

This patient desires to have the surgery done and get back to work.

However, she has been in a battle with her insurance company to

cover this surgical procedure. She has been to 3 different

orthopedists who all concur that the best treatment for her is to

have the hip replacement. The insurance company disagrees and

refuses to cover this surgery. She has been through all of their

pathways, including several courses of physical therapy, and is just

not getting better. Of course, she is no longer working so paying out

of pocket is impossible. And, she now requires the use of narcotic

pain medications to sleep at night, putting her at the risk of tolerance and dependence. While the insurance company is trying to cut costs, it is clear to see that is not happening here. It is creating other medical conditions in this patient that will likely be costly down the road. And, she is on disability through the state. The longer she is disabled, the more the state will be paying. It would make much more financial sense to fix her hip and get her back in the workplace. The most shocking thing about this case is that it started over 2 years ago. How many years does she have to suffer before the insurance company covers her the way they are supposed to?

There is little oversight to these denied care cases. The Insurance Commissioner can be asked to step in but that does not always go anywhere. And there are just too many cases happening that it would be impossible. So, what can one do when a needed test or surgery is denied? File an appeal. The patient can do this or the physician can do this. I have seen little luck on either side. And the decision of an appeal can take several weeks. If a patient is covered by an employer's plan, it sometimes helps to go to the HR department. But, really, why are all these steps needed?

Another big area where denied care is playing a bigger role is with prescription medications. In the past few months, I have had several asthmatic patients come to me wheezing because their generic inhalers are no longer covered under their prescription drug plan. These inhalers typically cost over $70 and are not easily affordable for many patients. These patients also did not receive any obvious notice that their coverage was changing. For asthmatics, inhalers are life-saving medications. Yet, these patients were made to wait days to weeks waiting for authorizations to be determined by their insurance companies.

And it is not only the expensive prescription brand name drugs that are being denied. I am seeing this increasingly with generic medications. For example, doxycycline which used to be on many stores $4 dollar plans is no longer covered and now costing over $70 out-of-pocket expenses at many pharmacies. How did the cost of this medication change so drastically? And I am seeing this with Prednisone as well.

Pharmaceutical companies are another large source of healthcare spending. Medications are expensive. So much so that many times patients simply go without taking them. I have seen many patients have to choose between two needed medications because they could not afford to take them both. Sometimes, I see patients who ran out of their blood pressure medications but cannot fill them until payday. Money needs to be spent on research and developing new drugs. No one would argue with that. However, if you look at the profits of the pharmaceutical companies you can see that Big Pharma is a big money-making business. If you buy the same medication in other countries, it would cost significantly less. For example, I was in Egypt one summer and needed an antibiotic. A 10 day course of Augmentin cost me the equivalent of $4. Here, patients typically tell me the cost is near or over $100 for the same duration. Of course, production costs are higher in the US. But, those big profits the pharmaceutical companies are making represent a big proportion of medication costs. It saddens me that my patients cannot afford the medications they need.

Inside Our Broken Healthcare System

I treated a patient recently who was experiencing some chest discomfort. It was not an acute problem, like a heart attack, that required the patient to go to the hospital. Rather, my medical decision was to do a nuclear stress test. However, her insurance company refused saying that according to their treatment guidelines, she was only eligible for a regular

exercise stress test. While I understand that this is a much less expensive option and suffices in most cases, this particular patient suffers from severe osteoarthritis of both knees and is simply unable to walk on a treadmill. Of course, the decision was appealed with this information and the prior authorization was rejected. A test to diagnose a cardiac problem in a patient to prevent a life-threatening cardiac complication, even death, resulted in a month long battle. I eventually decided to refer the patient to a cardiologist, who also went to battle and eventually won. So, what ended up being a cost-cutting measure on behalf of the insurance company ended up costing much more by the insistence of those with no real knowledge of a given patient making medical decisions.

How does denied care harm patients?

- When diagnostic tests are not done promptly, it leads to delayed, and even worse, missed diagnoses. You can see from the example of my lady with the chest discomfort. If she did have a significant cardiac problem, she could have had a fatal event while waiting for a prior authorization.

- And so, prompt treatment is not started when it is necessary. If someone has a disc herniation impinging on the spinal cord, it is imperative to consider surgery early to prevent permanent nerve damage. Yet, a MRI of the L-S spine is often one of the most difficult tests to be approved. It can take weeks and many phone calls. A patient just does not have weeks to stave off permanent harm.

- Alternatively, less costly medications are not always the best. I always try to keep costs in consideration when I write a prescription and most of my prescriptions are for generics. However, there are exceptions where the patient needs the more expensive medication. A good example of this can be seen in my COPD patients. Often, it is just trying to find the right inhaler that helps them be able to breathe. Most do fine with generics. But, there are some who simply do not respond except to the newer brand name medications. Often, time is taken to get prior-authorization of these medications and often it is just rejected. These patients suffer from not being able to get the medications they need.

- Sometimes insurance companies will change their formularies (the medications they will pay for). Often, my patients with GERD or gastritis will be required to change their medications based on a formulary change. They may have been doing well on their current medication for years. Yet, the insurance company does not consider this. Many of these patients will change against their wishes and end up having a return of their symptoms because of this change in medication. And then, the prior authorization war will begin again. I am seeing this in my hypertensive patients as well. Many companies have changed the medications covered on their formularies. I am seeing many patients with elevated blood pressures because of this.

- When patients are forced to accept these changes, distrust enters into the system. They start to hate healthcare and those involved in it. They tend to avoid coming for care unless it is absolutely necessary. And it is, at those times, that their medical conditions are in a much worse state.

- It drives a wedge in the doctor-patient relationship. Patients often do not see the great effort doctors undertake on their behalf to get their needed services covered. They do not believe that doctors are working on their behalf and the truth is often far from this. If you ask the patient how much time the doctor spent with them, they will answer a few minutes. They do not see the battles we fight for them behind the scenes. Denied tests and medications are becoming an all too frequent part of the out-patient medicine landscape. It is ironic that while they purport to cut costs, they often end up driving up costs by unneeded referrals to specialists and unnecessary ER visits. While it doesn't achieve its cost-cutting goal, the worse complication of this policy is the harm it causes patients. Doctors are not sitting in the exam room devising ways to cost the insurance company as much money as possible. We are not wantonly ordering tests just for the joy of it. When I order a test for a patient, there is a medical reason for my doing so. I have spent years in education and training to be able to examine and evaluate a patient and form a differential diagnosis. I have also been fully trained how to evaluate patients and diagnose dangerous diseases which should be ruled out. There is no way that a doctor or other healthcare worker sitting behind a desk without seeing or examining my patient can know what is better for the patient. Health insurance companies need to stop practicing medicine and rendering medical decisions on unseen patients. Patients deserve much better care than this. And many of them are paying for the cost to be insured out of their own pockets. It is truly disheartening when I have to tell a patient that the

insurance will not cover a test I think is medically necessary

for them.

Chapter 4: Understaffed Hospitals

Hospitals have shared in the financial crisis of medicine. Many smaller ones have simply closed their doors or consolidated with larger ones. Additionally, many hospitals have had to cut support staff to stay afloat. It is often in the higher paid employees, such as RN's, where the cuts are made to reduce costs. Less skilled staff is tasked with filling that void and patients have been feeling this.

I had recently had a patient tell me that they rang their call bell 3 times over an hour period to ask for their ordered pain medications. And this was a post-surgical patient.

A study of California hospitals showed that ER patients have a higher risk of dying if a nearby ER closed its doors shortly before. In recent years, 6% of ERs have stopped operating. In contrast, visits to ERs have increased by 51%, leading to over-crowding and longer waits. After adjusting for different hospital and patient characteristics, the researchers found that inpatients at hospitals affected by closures were 5% more likely to die than patients at other hospitals. The risk for those below 65 years of age was even greater (10% higher than those inpatients in other hospitals). When they looked at heart attack, stroke and sepsis patients, they had a mortality rate 15% higher at hospitals with nearby ER closures than at other hospitals. The reason appears to be multifactorial. Some suggest that the longer distance to the next closest ER plays a factor. Overcrowding and longer wait times also appear to play a significant role. Still others suggest that patients put off seeking care because of this and thus arrive in worse shape. 1

In the first quarter of 2014, seven hospitals filed for bankruptcy. 2 And we can expect this problem to get worse as hospitals struggle to get paid and comply with increasing regulations and mandates. Regarding patient complaints about quality of care in hospitals, I am hearing these all too frequently. How many times have you heard of a patient on a bed pan for over half an hour waiting for someone to come to their aid? This is becoming a common occurrence. And this has nothing to do with the nurses not caring. Nurses do care but they are over-worked and do not have enough hands available.

There is only so much they can do and they try their best. Patients are often commenting on the "old days" and having nurses care for them at their bedside. Nurses just don't have the time these days. With all the cuts in hospital staff, more and more is expected of them and they have less and less coworkers to assist them. Another place where this is readily evident is in our countries' emergency departments. We all hear about the 5-6 hour waits to be treated. Some of this is a symptom of our broken system and the fact that these patients really do not belong in the ER. However, ER's are simply not staffed to handle this volume of patients. And we can expect this to get worse as the physician shortage expands.

How are understaffed hospitals harming patients?

- When staff is overworked and overwhelmed, errors can occur. The same is true for anyone in any profession. Hospital cuts have resulted in hospitals cutting back on staff causing the remaining workers to have to pick up the slack of those who were cut.

- When there are not enough hands around, patients have to wait for care. One nurse can simply do so much. Nurses are truly inspiring workers and do so much good in the healthcare field. But, they are human too. They are expected to do too many tasks these days. This can lead to frustration and burnout.

- Patients start to distrust hospitals. I hear so many patients who simply do not want to go to the hospital for any reason. This is a very dangerous situation because they put off emergency care when it is needed. I recently was seeing a gentleman with chest pain. His EKG showed cardiac ischemia and I thought he may be having a heart attack. He was initially refusing to go to the hospital because he "hated" hospitals. After much argument, he finally agreed. He went and was indeed diagnosed with an acute myocardial infarction. If he went home instead of the ER, he may have died. Everyone knows time is of the essence when treating a heart attack. However, many patients remember bad experiences from prior ER visits or hospital admissions and do not wish to return, even when obviously needed.

- There becomes a strained relationship between the patients and nurses. I hear many patients tell me while they were in the hospital that the nurse did not care about them. I tell them they care much more than the patient will ever know and they are just very over-worked these days.

- Hospitals now have less trained staff doing more specialized jobs. The role of the RN has been delegated to less LPN's and even medical assistants, who have less training. In any job, especially where lives are at stake, it is always best to have the most highly trained people doing the job for which they are skilled. Like with anything else, less trained people just will not be able to do the same quality job as the person who possesses the skills and training to do it.

There are approximately 2.5 million nurses in the US. In a recent survey, it was found that nurses are overworked and stressed out. In fact 89% of those surveyed feel that they cannot do their jobs adequately because their supervisors don't care and they lack support staff. Nurses are so overworked and stressed that 64% rarely get 7-8 hours of sleep per night and 77% responded that they do not eat well regularly. Hospitals are now underfunded and nurses are doing more than their fair share of work. Yet, only 16% of those who answered felt that they were adequately compensated. 3 Nurses are on the frontlines and put themselves at risk every day for the sake of their patients. They deserve better than this. In one study, more than 1/3 of nurses reported being burnt out. And this was shown to increase hospital infection rates. In this study, researchers looked at approximately 7,000 nurses in over 161 hospitals. They looked specifically at the rate of urinary catheter infections. They found that: "Nurses had an average patient load of 5.7 patients. For every additional patient assigned to a nurse, there was about one extra catheter-associated urinary tract infection per 1,000 patients. And when hospitals have 10 percent more burnt-out nurses, there was an additional one catheter-associated infection and two additional surgical site infections per 1,000 patients." 4

Understaffing does not just happen at the level of nurses. Many hospitalists are now shouldering extra work. In a recent survey, 36% of hospitalists reported carrying an unsafe patient load more than once a week. It was felt that these unsafe workloads led to poor communication, unsafe turn-over of the patients, medical mistakes, unnecessary tests being ordered, and sometimes even medical complications. 5

Another area where hospital understaffing can have a very disastrous effect is in the operating room. One study looked at this in particular and found that understaffed ORs were the biggest threats to patient safety. It was felt that hospital staff is the last layer to detecting any errors that may affect patient safety. When there is not enough staff, that last layer of protection is missing and that is when errors sneak through. 6

Understaffed hospitals are a very real problem in the US healthcare system. As healthcare pushes to cut costs more, we can expect this problem to get worse. This is a threat to patient safety and prohibits quality of medical care. What is the point to have great workers when you just don't have enough hands to assist? And this is driving burnout among these professionals who are expected to be empathetic and caring. No one should be so stressed out by their chosen profession that they don't sleep or eat right. The role doctors and nurses play in the hospital is truly a valuable, irreplaceable one. Unless we start treating them right and getting enough staff on deck, we will find many of them leaving the hospital setting. These workers are putting themselves on the frontlines for the sake of caring for patients and deserve to be more respected. When a patient goes to the hospital, it is because they are going through a very serious illness or injury. They should be

cared for and receive the attention they deserve. Unless this

problem is addressed, we are facing a real crisis of medical care in

hospitals.

1- http://www.cnn.com/2014/08/05/health/emergency-room-closures/

2- http://www.beckershospitalreview.com/eweekly/HRE040 314.htm

3- http://www.healthline.com/health-news/nurses-overworked-understaffed-070714

4- http://www.fiercehealthcare.com/story/nurse-burnout-understaffing-linked-hospital-infections/2012-07-30

5- http://www.medscape.com/viewarticle/778338?pa=oXNY Tnp5MqlHT43N3hEaUMt4uQlMx0p7UWXQNQppXR46LHizl vwFRFMS%2FzsUsvY6dewKyYGlndQjRAxd6xaO3Q%3D%3D

6- http://www.biomedcentral.com/1471-2482/12/10

Chapter 5: Over-regulation of Doctors

Inside Our Broken Healthcare System

Now, more than ever, new regulations and mandates are being placed on doctors. Patients may not necessarily feel this directly, but this is affecting patient care. We are spending more and more time, as well as dollars, to comply with this increased regulatory burden. We are simply stretched to the limit, yet more keeps being asked of us. We have new compliance guidelines to implement to ensure that   we are providing quality care. These are things that we have always been doing in our practices, but now are required to submit data proving it. This data was determined by non-physicians to be analyzed by non-physicians to determine whether we are providing acceptable care. Surely, if we are forced to comply with these new quality indicators, we should have some say in determining the quality.

Currently, it seems like new regulations are being made for doctors every day. While keeping up with these new mandates is burdensome for everyone, it is causing havoc on small practices. Unlike larger groups or hospitals, we just do not have the staff to implement all these changes. Nor can we afford it even if we wanted it. While many proclaim these new requirements, such as Meaningful Use, NCQA, e-prescribing, etc., are going to improve clinical outcomes, many doctors are just not seeing that reality. In fact, there is no evidence supporting that these mandates in fact improve clinical outcomes.

How are increasing mandates harmful?

– Doctors need to spend increasing time keeping up with these mandates. Unfortunately, we cannot do everything at the same time so we need to find this time from somewhere. Oftentimes, the only place left is the time we spend with patients. Patient diseases are becoming more complex and new treatments are proliferating. Is it better for a doctor to spend time learning the latest treatment options that can be offered to a patient, or to use that time learning which box to check so our metrics are adequately captured by the regulators?

– When these regulations become standard, often the thinking process goes out the window. For example, prior authorizations for diagnostic tests and medications are often decided by people who are not physicians and just following guidelines. Even when doctors appeal and state the reason why the patient needs a certain procedure or medication, it is often arbitrarily denied. Surely, some clinical reasoning should go into denials for services a doctor feels necessary for their patients. Additionally, doctors have been speaking up against Meaningful Use mandates. Many of us don't feel the EHR technology is there yet to be clinically useful. Yet, there are metrics in place that we need to record to prove we are using it meaningfully. This disconnect is also hazardous. Doctors need to be data entry clerks to record metrics that we don't feel beneficial to our patients. Is it better if doctors decide how to use their EHR for the best patient care? Do we truly need to document at every visit that an infant is a non-smoker?

– Implementing the necessary practice changes to keep in compliance is costly. Physicians are probably the only profession that does not receive cost of living increases to our salaries. Our reimbursements are shrinking or stagnating. Overhead costs are soaring. It is already very difficult to keep our doors open financially. Yet, this added burden is being cast around our necks. Isn't it better for doctors to invest in new services and technology for patient care rather than investing in metrics recording technology for insurance companies?

– In small practices, staff needs to take on the role of doing this additional work. They too are only human and can do so much. They need to take time away from other tasks to accomplish the requirements set forth. This too is time taken away from patients. Wouldn't it be better for the staff in a doctor's office to concentrate on patients?

While data can be a good thing, when it goes over-board it can have the opposite effect of what was intended. We all want improved clinical outcomes. And the spirit of some of these requirements is not all bad. But, when the regulations become the primary goal, patient care will suffer. It is time to put the patient back in the spotlight. They are the ones we are all working for. It is time to make regulations that are clinically useful and focus on the patient.

And maybe it is time to put doctors in charge of that task rather than executives and politicians.

One sign of the way these regulations is overly burdensome and unreasonable can be seen with the use of EHRS and the meaningful use program.

Many patients come to me stating that the other doctor didn't listen to them, that they were just interested in looking in their computers the whole visit. Patients don't realize why. We are no longer just responsible for documenting their office visit for the sake of having a record available to provide medical care for them. We are required to document certain metrics in order to comply with the Meaningful Use program. And most of the technology that currently exists has not been evolved to the place where doctors find that its use is meaningful for clinical practice. As more medical records go digital, many end users (i.e. doctors) are growing increasingly frustrated with the state of their electronic health record (EHR) system. Various polls have shown a majority of doctors find EHRs slow them down and don't easily adapt to their workflow, and they also feel EHR developers do not truly understand how EHRs are being used. The technology has not been created to fit our needs, yet we're mandated to use it in order to qualify for meaningful use (MU).

While MU is currently an incentive program, it will in the future be used to penalize doctors who do not comply. I don't think anyone would argue about the value of EHRs, especially if they are ever to achieve any significant degree of interoperability. They have a huge potential to improve outcomes and save lives. For example, if a patient arrives in the ER in the middle of the night from a drug overdose, anyone can see the value of the ER physician being able to log into that patient's medical records to be able to determine what drug/medication he may have taken. But, that kind of interoperability is far in the future. Interfaces between current systems are proving difficult and are often incompatible.

How do doctors need EHRs to evolve?

1. EHRs need to be customized to a doctor's workflow to help improve efficiency. As it is now, they are a time drain, slowing doctors down and forcing many to chart after hours as a result.

2. Vendors need to understand the needs of the doctor and adapt their products to fit better. Currently, the software is developed and the physician is forced to try to make it work – this often fails.

3. Test results should be more easily uploaded into systems. For example, pulmonary function tests, EKGs, Holtor monitors, or any test which a doctor gets results on computer software should integrate with the practice's EHR system. Ours does not, forcing us to download it and then upload it. We have to print EKGs out and scan them into the chart. Not only is this another time drain, it increases the chance for errors to creep into the system. For example, results can be uploaded into wrong files.

4. Interfaces should be a priority. The interfaces we built with Quest and Labcorp took approximately eight months to complete. These are two of the biggest labs in the country and, if they had problems, what happens with smaller labs? Adding to the frustration: our hospital was never able to interface with our system.

5. Notes need to return to being readable for patient care. As it is now, when we request a note, we will get six to seven pages of minutia and have to dig out the relevant medical facts. Much of this has to do with the fact that EHRs were designed more with billing purposes in mind – something we already know how to do. We need a record that is medically relevant to treat patients effectively.

6. EHRs should be easily accessible from outside our practice. Now, I use LogMeIn but this often wastes time as well. If there was a HIPAA-compliant function that made it easy to access our own records at any time, that would really help save time and improve patient care. Everyone is talking about telemedicine

these days, but wouldn't telemedicine work better if we could easily access medical records?

7. Systems should be easily customizable. Practices change. I do procedures today that I didn't do three or four years ago. The EHR needs to adapt to changes in practice, and updates should be easy to perform. When I do my quarterly software update, I have to turn off all the work stations to do it. This is disruptive. Many good things come from an EHR implementation, from improved patient care to more organized notes. EHRs can greatly improve our tracking systems and insure all our patients get needed tests done and that they return for follow up when they should. It is much more efficient doing this with EHRs than with paper charts and, when systems truly become interoperable, healthcare throughout the medical ecosystem will improve. But, to get there, much work and evolution is still needed. And unless you include the end users in the discussion and development, chances are that this is more a dream than a reality. **EHRs are not the revolutionary tools that they are**

claimed to be. What happens when the system goes down? We once had our system go down for 3 days. In that time, we had no access to our schedule, patient charts, blood work results, x-ray reports or billing data. We had to see our patients without all of this. Sure, paper charts get misplaced. But, it does not compare with an electronic system failure. There is still much work to be done to improve the software.

Interoperability is another bone of contention. EHRs were supposed to be interoperable, that is interface with other systems, labs and hospitals so that a patient's medical records are always available. But, they failed on this front. Interoperability seems to be the key word in health IT these days. Those of us in the healthcare field dream of a day when we have true interoperability across systems. A day, that is, when we can access the patient's data wherever that may be, with the use of our own systems.

Inside Our Broken Healthcare System

Many people say physicians are reluctant to adapt new technology and this reluctance is keeping us from reaching the goal of true interoperability. But, the reality is the technology is just not there yet. In my own practice, I have struggled to make my own systems interoperable. My EHR software's support team has been trying to interface with my web site to make my patient portal active for eight months and have been unable to do so. This inability to interface creates extra steps for my staff and wastes time – time that could be spent doing something more productive. It also leads to the possibility of a patient's information being erroneously filed into another patient's chart. Needless to say, the problems my staff is experiencing are not acceptable, nor is the inconvenience I encounter when I'm in the exam room with a patient and do not have his results available because they were sitting in the scanning queue waiting to be filed. When my staff or I call support, we are always told that our interface is at the top of their priority list. Nevertheless, there is no estimation of when this interfacing will be completed. Our EHR has interfaced with two large labs - Quest and Labcorp — but smaller labs have tried to interface and were unable. The hospitals in my area, as well as radiology facilities near me, do not have the capabilities to interface with my EHR, so for now, we are logging into their individual websites, downloading test results, and pasting them into a patient's chart. A second option is to receive the results by fax and scan them into record. While we long for ease of access of patient data through a completely operable infrastructure, the technology still does not support this. We need to call on EHR vendors to step up the technology to allow the interfacing that needs to be done to make our systems communicate with each other. As it stands now, there are numerous EHR vendors out there making it overwhelmingly difficult for a provider to know which one is best. For now, we have to wait for the technology to catch up to our aspirations. But once this happens, the ability to interface and communicate between systems will make us more efficient and save time, freeing us up to spend more time with our patients. It also should decrease the risk of results being misfiled. Mandates surrounding EHRs use at this point just make no sense. Perhaps, the EHRs themselves need to be mandated and regulated before this burden is pushed onto doctors.

PQRS is another mandate that has been placed upon physicians by CMS. Under this program, physicians are required to submit certain metrics for various diseases, such as diabetes, to Medicare along with billing data. This reporting is labor intensive and the guidelines confusing and difficult to follow. There are minimum numbers of patients required and some doctors just don't have that volume. Many doctors did not participate because we honestly do not have time. I much rather spend my time with my diabetic patients counseling them on their diets than recording data about their labs to be harvested by Medicare. My patients prefer that as well. Starting in 2015, any provider who did not submit the data will be fined 1% of their reimbursements. This fine is expected to increase yearly. Many doctors simply are at their breaking point. Many are choosing to opt out of the Medicare program rather than persist under these burdensome mandates and face the penalties. This is going to create a true problem of access for seniors as more physicians choose to opt-out.

ICD10 is another area where there is much debate. It is a whole new system of coding office visits to submit for billing purposes. It is a very confusing and labor intensive system. We are currently using ICD9 and this by itself is time consuming. There have been instances where I spent more time looking up a certain code than I actually spent with the patient. Its proponents claim that it will improve clinical outcomes. But, in reality, it is just a tool for the usefulness to insurance companies. It serves no good purpose in patient care. Again, there is no good evidence that it will improve clinical outcomes for patients.

Another mandate that is consuming doctors' time is complying with the new **MOC** (Maintenance of Certification) process. Doctors are becoming increasingly vocal over a system that we are forced to partake in and feel there is no benefit for us. It is costly and has turned into a profitable business for the medical boards and their members.

Why do doctors think the MOC requirements are unfair?

1. We do not feel like we are being tested on what is relevant to clinical medicine. We should be tested on things that are needed to be known to competently perform our medical duties.

2. We are required to pay thousands of dollars to be in the MOC process. There are some doctors who claim this is nothing more than a money-making idea for the boards.

3. We are already required to do a certain number of CME hours to maintain our medical licenses. In order to meet the number of hours required, doctors read educational materials and attend conferences. These keep us informed on the latest updates in medicine. Often, the tests are asking questions on outdated guidelines.

4. Many states require physicians to do CME hours in certain areas. For example, in NJ, we are required to complete CME hours in cultural competency. We have many immigrants in our state. This is a great way to ensure we are keeping up on a needed area of focus. Other states have required CME hours in HIV, domestic violence, etc.

5. The MOC modules are very time-consuming. They are not something that can be completed during a work day. We need to take several hours of personal time to complete these. And most of us feel these modules add little value in terms of practical knowledge. In essence, we are being forced to pay for educational activities that most of us feel are worthless.

6. Board certification is required to be on staff at most hospitals as well as to be contracted with most insurance plans. Some may claim that MOC/board certification is voluntary. However, we are excluded from participating in insurance plans and being able to have hospital privileges if we do not comply. Thus, we are forced to follow the MOC requirements to maintain our practice of medicine

and be able to get paid for our services.

7. Many of the people who are developing the requirements are not practicing physicians. Thus, they are not qualified to assess the skill of those practicing clinically. Yet, much of the MOC process has been devised by those not practicing medicine or are even doctors. Doctors should be evaluated on a regular basis to determine they are competent to safely treat physicians. However, most physicians feel that the MOC requirements are not the way to do it and are more a forced activity that adds to our costs with little useful benefit to us. Perhaps, CME could be better reported to serve our needs and ensure our skills. Or perhaps, physicians can be asked to devise a way their colleagues' level of competency be determined. They are, after all, the only ones who truly know what needs to be known and done to treat patients once they step inside that exam room. While life-long learning is a necessity in the medical field, MOC is not the way to achieve it. Clearly, a better model needs to be developed. And physicians need to be key advisees. It is taking time away from our patients in order to fulfill these requirements.

Inside Our Broken Healthcare System

Medicine is rapidly advancing and doctors need to stay current with all the new technology out there, from robotics to new medications to genomic studies. While we are trying to keep abreast of all these advancements, new mandates and regulations are being imposed on us. Often these are determined by government employees or big insurance companies. Neither of these agencies have anyone to answer to. They can pass these mandates and we just have to comply. It is taking our focus away from where it should be: patient care. This is no longer acceptable. Any new mandate should undergo intense scrutiny and have the input of practicing physicians. It is not alright to force us to purchase inferior technology to meet these regulations. Overhaul the EHR and health IT industries first. Make them show quality products and get input from doctors to be sure it is matching what we need in the exam room.

As it stands, these regulations are dumbing down medicine and enslaving us to do work that we disagree with. As a physician, I would much rather put my efforts into face to face time with my patients and invest in technology that has a direct effect on

improving the quality of medical care for my patients.

Chapter 6: Malpractice Crisis

Inside Our Broken Healthcare System

We live in a lawsuit friendly society. Everyone looks to cast blame when something goes wrong. Have you ever been in an automobile accident? Then you know that the police report is public record and soon followed by an onslaught of letters from lawyers trying to represent you in filing a claim for your injuries. Where there is a bad outcome, people are looking for someone to blame. Often, the finger is pointed to the doctor and the medical team.   The realization that every procedure has the possibility of a bad outcome despite the best possible care goes unrecognized. This is despite the fact that patients sign consent forms explaining all the risks of a given procedure and confirming that they are aware of these possible bad outcomes. They just never believe that it can happen to them. And since it is expected in only a small percentage of cases, surely something wrong must have been done. But, most often, this is not the case.

According to the AMA, more than 61% of doctors over the age of 55 years have been sued at least one. Approximately, 10-20% of cases occur because of a missed diagnosis. The malpractice litigation hits some specialties harder than others. For example, general surgeons and OB/GYN doctors tend to be sued the most. Almost 70% of doctors in these specialties have been sued at least once and 50% have been sued 2 or more times. The least likely to be sued are pediatricians and psychiatrists. While there are a large number of suits, few of these results in any payments and doctors most often win the cases when they go to court. Most cases never make it to the court room but are rather settled prior to going to trial. In 2012, payouts from lost malpractice cases resulted in payouts of $3.6 billion. 1

It is not just the direct effect of litigation that drives up healthcare costs. A recent Gallop poll showed that approximately 1 out of every 4 healthcare dollars goes into defensive medicine.   An independent healthcare economics firm, BioScience Valuation, estimates the annual cost of defensive medicine exceeds $480 billion. RAND corporation reported that 3 states adapted tort reform hoping to show a reduction in healthcare spending that ERs spend towards defensive medication. They failed to show any difference. 2

Malpractice suits are damaging in many ways, not just to a physician's reputation. It causes untold stress upon the physician being sued and contributes to burnout. The less burnout that is present, the better a doctor will be. These suits take countless hours and takes time away from face-to-face patient care. It also harms the doctor- patient relationship, not just with the patient filing the lawsuit. When a doctor is sued for unreasonable cause, they begin to distrust their patients. The doctor-patient relationship is one based on trust, going both ways. The more the trust, the stronger the relationship will be.

I know many OB/GYN doctors have stopped delivering babies because they are no longer able to afford their malpractice premium payments. The risk of being sued for delivery a baby with problems has gotten to be too costly for many doctors. This is harmful because we are decreasing our pool of available OB/GYN doctors. While everyone is saddened when a baby has complications, there is often no way to prevent them from happening. Yet, this represents a big area of liability. I know of one

OB/Gyn who lost everything after being sued. At the time the suit

was filed, her malpractice carrier filed for bankruptcy. This

essentially left her uninsured. She lost her home and most of her

savings in this suit. And she was not even the primary obstetrician

in the delivery of this baby. She was just on-call and covering for

another physician. The delivery was uneventful yet, the baby was

born with cerebral palsy. As physicians, we know that not all cases

of CP result from birth trauma. Sometimes, despite the best

medical care, babies are born with this disease and there is no way

to prevent it. Yet, doctors are often found liable for babies born

with CP, whether they are at fault or not. She no longer delivers

babies although she is a fine doctor.

I once had a patient threaten to sue me for refusing to prescribe a

narcotic pain medication for her. She was a new patient to me and I

had no records for her. In my area, it is not uncommon to see

patients who "doctor shop", looking for many doctors just to give them prescriptions for controlled substances. She raised many red

flags in my mind. No doctor should be threatened for going against

their better judgment. We should not feel pressured to practice

medicine under the threat of litigation. For one thing, it drives up

healthcare costs for unnecessary care. And it is just bad medicine

and not in the best interests of our patients. Yet, these types of

stories are happening frequently all across the country. Patients

need protection from malpractice and medical negligence but it

must be a fair process. It has strayed far from its intended course.

Doctors can be sued for any reason without any evidence of wrong-

doing. Jury decisions are often decided by emotional factors and

not medical facts. While everyone is trying to cure the problem of

the uninsured and the burden they place on our healthcare system,

there will be no healthcare reform without tort reform.

How can we achieve relevant tort reform in the healthcare system?

- One thing that can be considered is a system of arbitration rather than taking these cases through the judicial system.

- We need to eliminate frivolous lawsuits. These drive up liability costs and serve no useful purpose.

- The loser in a malpractice case should pay the litigation costs. This is a way to ensure that only serious cases are brought to trial.

- Verdicts in malpractice cases should be decided by a jury of peers, meaning medical professionals, not the general public. This would help ensure that outcomes are determined by medical facts and not emotion.

- There should be financial caps on awards.

Our litigious society is contributory to the high healthcare costs in the US. One quarter of healthcare dollars has been estimated to go towards the practice of defensive medicine. Many studies are ordered out of fear of liability. When we see that the majority of lawsuits are filed because of missed diagnoses, it is easy to understand this. Malpractice premiums have gone through the roof and many doctors are struggling to pay them. If this upward trend continues, some doctors may soon stop performing high risk procedures. We are already seeing this in the field of OB/GYN where many doctors have stopped delivering babies because of the malpractice risk. We are losing many highly skilled doctors because of this. Tort reform needs to be addressed if we truly want healthcare reform. It is another symptom of our broken healthcare system. Doctors should be able to practice good medicine without the threat of lawsuit always hanging over their heads. Sure, patients need remedy if they have been faulted. But, the medical malpractice system has over-stepped its bounds. Do we want doctors providing the best medical treatments for our patients because we care about them? Or would we rather doctors who practice to avoid litigation?

1- http://www.physicianspractice.com/blog/ten-notable-physician-related-malpractice-statistics

2- http://www.forbes.com/sites/theapothecary/2014/11/05/dont-reform-the-malpractice-system-to-reduce-healthcare-costs-eliminate-it/2/

Chapter 7: Physician Shortage

For years, experts have been predicting a physician shortage. Well, we are now there and it is only going to get worse. The area I practice has been declared a primary care shortage area by the AAFP (American Academy of Family Physicians). Patients have a hard time locating a primary care provider and it can take weeks to get an appointment. This is despite the fact that many insurance companies require them to have a PCP (primary care physician) before receiving any other medical care.   And this shortage is only going to get worse for many reasons. For one thing, there is an influx of newly insured patients under the ACA. This comes with no increase in the number of trained physicians. More doctors are retiring earlier or changing careers and there has been a shift away from primary care in recent years. Soon, we will see a true crisis of healthcare access like exists in other countries. It has been estimated that by 2020, there will be a shortage of 90,000 physicians. By 2025, it is estimated that there will be a shortage of 140,000 physicians. Complicating this fact is that 1 in 3 physicians is over 55 years of age and close to retirement. While the supply of

doctors is dwindling, the demand is increasing. There are about

10,000 people who turn 65 every day. By the age of 65 years, 2/3

of people have at least one chronic medical condition. Of all the

patients over 65 years, approximately 20% see 14 or more

physicians each year. And there has been no increase in the

number of physicians being trained. Medicare-sponsored residency

slots have been capped since 1997. And it is expected that medical

graduates will soon outnumber residency slots. It is felt that this

shortage is no longer restricted to primary care but extends across

several specialties. 1

What will happen because of the physician shortage?

-It will be more difficult for a patient to schedule an appointment

and there will be a longer wait to get on the schedule.

- Elective procedures will take months to get scheduled.

- Referrals to specialists will require longer waiting periods.

Depending on the specialty, it may take months to get in to see a specialist. I am already seeing this in some cases.

- It will be harder to be treated by an MD/DO. Patients will be forced to see mid-level providers who are less trained.

-Patients will put off getting diagnostic tests because of the long waits. People have busy lives. It is hard to schedule anything weeks or months down the road.

- Diseases will be diagnosed at more advanced stages because of this access of care crisis. For years, experts have predicted a physician shortage, especially in the primary care fields. Little has been done to increase the number of physicians choosing to pursue these specialties or increase the number of doctors to fill the gap.

- Rather, some are calling for mid-level providers to step up and fill this deficiency. While mid-levels can greatly assist and are much-needed in primary care, they are still not physicians and will not fill the gap. While they can work unsupervised in some states, in others they can only work under a physician's supervision.

Why Mid-Levels Will Not Fill The Primary Care Gap?

— Their training is different. They are educated and trained to be mid-levels, Doctors are educated and trained to be doctors. They are not interchangeable. They are a great asset, but they are not trained to be doctors and should not be used to replace doctors.

— Many patients prefer being treated by physicians. While I have nothing against a patient who would rather see a mid-level provider than me, the patient should have enough options to be able to choose who they would like to see. They should not be forced to be treated by a mid-level because there are just not any physicians available for them. And, in the final analysis, we are all working for good outcomes for the patients and helping them be their own advocates.

— Mid-levels are not as well as trained to treat high risk patients. Many people have stated that the increased number of mid-levels will result in doctors seeing the high risk patients. But, as the population ages, so does the number of high risk patients. There will be many more complicated patients resulting from increasing age, the rising incidence of obesity, diabetes mellitus and other chronic diseases. The number of physicians needs to be increased to match these needs.

– Mid-levels still need to call on physicians when they have questions. While they can see and treat patients, in some states without supervision, they still need doctors available as back up. Doctors are already overwhelmed by the increasing number of patients and demands being placed on us. Not all of us have any time left to supervision the growing number of mid-levels now practicing. While mid-levels can help ease the looming physician shortage, they are not going to fill the void. More doctors are still going to be needed. As more patients are being insured under the ACA, more doctors need to be available. To provide the highest quality care, a team approach needs to be taken. Mid-levels provide a valuable service to medicine and are highly competent to treat many medical conditions. But, they still cannot replace doctors. As more and more patients become insured, as patients age and more complex medical problems are seen, we are still going to need more physicians. Yet, the number of physicians being educated and trained has not increased very much in recent years. While an individual doctor may feel overwhelmed and overworked by the shortage, the true crisis is the lack of access. This will be felt most by the ones we are all trying to help: the patient. Unless the number of residency trained positions is increased, we will soon be facing a crisis of access in our healthcare system.

1- http://www.beckershospitalreview.com/hospital-physician-relationships/8-physician-shortage-statistics.html

Chapter 8: Isolation

It is illegal for doctors to unionize or collectively bargain. For this reason, many doctors feel completely isolated from others. While we see many ills in our healthcare system and grow weary of trying to give our patients the best while fighting the system, it is just too hard to do so individually. Many times the doctor who speaks out gets labeled disruptive. As doctors, we are getting more disenchanted with our chosen profession. And rarely, are we asked to give a voice on how to repair it.

Why is physician isolation bad?

- We need to collaborate with other doctors to keep up with the latest treatments and technologies. Sure, we can read about them. But, it is much more beneficial hearing real world experience and how other doctors are using these things.

- Mandates are being poured on our heads and we are overwhelmed in keeping up and complying with them. As the ones on the frontlines of medicine, we need to be the ones to shape them. We cannot do this in isolation. We need to speak with other doctors to enable us to get our collective voice out.

- Technology in medicine is advancing like never before. We need input from our colleagues in shaping our technology goals.

- By being isolated, doctors are being taken advantage of. We need to find a way to come together and fight back.

- The rate of depression, burnout and suicide among physicians is rising.

Doctor burnout is a rising phenomenon in the field of medicine. More is expected of doctors these days than ever before. There are new medical discoveries being made virtually every day. In addition to staying educated on these new findings, there are unique governmental regulations being rolled out all too frequently. These include meaningful use, PQRS, certified medical homes and others, which are all very time consuming and labor intensive. At the same time, insurance companies have required increasing amounts of paperwork and bureaucracy.

What is contributing to physician burnout?

– As stated above, rapidly advancing technologies and discoveries in medicine that we are expected to be aware of.

– Increased regulatory burdens from the government and insurance companies.

– Decreasing or stagnating incomes that do not adjust for rising overhead expenses or cost of living increases.

– Increased liability issues. This problem continues to flourish allowing unneeded stress to be the backbone of much of what we do. Without tort reform and eliminating frivolous lawsuits, it will continue unchecked. Doctors pay high malpractice insurance premiums and many times feel much of medicine is done for defensive reasons.

– Increased denial of care is also a cause of our burnout. Increasingly, insurance companies are denying tests that doctors consider are medically necessary. Prescribed medications are often not covered by patients' prescription coverage. This is leading to an increasing feeling of helplessness among doctors. We are trying to offer our patients the best medical care possible. Yet, often we feel our hands are tied by the insurance companies.

– Patients are increasingly unhappy. They are forced to buy their own premiums and facing higher deductibles which they have to pay out-of-pocket. Frustration creeps in when they are unable to get the tests done that their doctor prescribed or take medications that they need.

– Life/work balance has become unbalanced. Doctors are working more hours than ever before. We are expected to take calls at night, on weekends and holidays. These are services that we often do not get paid to do. Yet, many patients have no appreciation of this. It has become an expectation.

– Lack of solidarity among physicians. We often feel isolated and alone in our struggles. We do not see that other doctors are facing the same struggles that we are. This leads to isolation.

We are facing increasing changes in the healthcare field. Many physicians feel that we are expected to give more and more while we are getting less and less. This overwhelms many doctors leading to burnout. And many of these factors are completely out of our control. We feel trapped in a system that we feel is not working and is in fact broken. We have little voice to speak up against many of the injustices we are seeing in this system. These feelings lead to burnout. More doctors are looking for alternative careers or to retire early. Many physicians are finding little enjoyment in their chosen profession. We need to get back to the system where doctors have a voice about what happens in medicine. A system where patients get the care they deserve. Isolation also leads to depression among physicians

In fact, it has been estimated that 300-400 physicians commit suicide every year. 1   Doctors are expected to be strong. We are not expected to show any signs of weakness. This depression coupled with isolation often proves deadly. The rate of physician suicide has not been decreasing. It is an often over-looked and neglected topic.

How do we disrupt this physician isolation?

- Our medical societies need to throw out politics and start to speak up for its physician members.
- Doctors no longer have time to spend in the doctors' lounge. We need a return of this place where we can have informal discussions with each other.
- We need to step up as teachers and shape the next generation of doctors. We need to help fix the system so they do not inherit this brokenness.
- We need to be leaders. It is no longer OK to just sit on the sidelines and complain.
- We need to leverage social media to these goals

Medical advances are happening at a seemingly break neck speed. Technology has greatly eased many tasks in our daily lives at work, at home and socially. It has also made it more difficult in some aspects. There is more we need to learn and know how to use. This is true for everyone but especially physicians. Not only are new technologies being developed in the practice of medicine, such as robotics and nanotechnologies, but in the more mundane aspects of how we communicate with each other and with our patients. The population is aging and suffering more complicated diseases. Our knowledge of these diseases has grown exponentially, as well as the treatment options available. It has never been more important to be able to communicate with other physicians and to get information out that is easily accessible for patients to learn about their disease processes and become advocates for themselves. Yet, 44% of physicians do not use social media at work and 60% use it for personal use only.

While it has been estimated that 90% of all adults in this country are using social media, 29% of doctors do not use it at all. Less than 30% use it for keeping up with medical news and/or interacting with peers. One of the reasons 23% of doctors cite for not using it is that they are not familiar with it. Other reasons include privacy concerns, time constraints, liability issues and the belief that there is no value in it. Another big concern for physicians is HIPAA concerns and there have been cases where doctors have gotten into trouble for this. Doctors are obviously lagging behind other fields in the use of social media. But, more and more doctors are finding the benefits of using these tools in medicine.

What are the benefits of using social media for physicians?

1. Clinical collaboration: Doctors are now able to communicate through social media channels. In earlier times, if we would want to get the opinion or help of a colleague, we would resort to attempting to contact them by phone or sending a written request. Social media has revolutionized the ways doctors can communicate with each other. Now, we are able to crowd-source. We can get more opinions in less time. Our colleagues are much more easily accessible and it can be done in real-time while we are treating a patient. We can use advanced technology to share things such as digital x-rays. These goals can be accomplished on various social media channels. Twitter is one example but it is sometimes hard to tweet to the doctors you need the information from. The best way to truly crowd source among colleagues is through online communities. You can share information in physician only communities that are not accessible to the public. Perhaps the best in this regards is **Sermo** (https://www.sermo.com) because it is

truly HIPAA compliant in that not only are the patients anonymous, the doctors are as well. It would be nearly impossible to trace a certain case back to a specific patient. Yet only 29% of doctors are using online physician communities.

2. Disseminating information for patients: A big task for doctors is educating our patients. We do this by giving written advice and handing out patient educational materials from various sources. Now, providing patients with educational materials is much easier. We can give them links to various websites that we feel beneficial. And we can disseminate general medical information through various channels: twitter, Facebook and blogging are good examples. There may be a day that it is reasonable for a doctor to communicate with their patients through social media platforms. However, at this stage, HIPAA greatly limits what we can do in this regards. But, we can direct a patient to a particular post we blogged or tweeted in order for them to get a greater understanding of their circumstances.

3. Medical Education between Physicians: As physicians, our

learning and studying never ends. We are required to get so many CME hours by our licensing boards. But, we also need to stay abreast of changes happening in our respective fields. We have been attending live events for ages. We can now attend teleconferences and webinars. Again, social media has changed the landscape in this regards. We now can have twitter chats amongst trusted colleagues around certain medical topics. And we can learn the latest medical news on social media sites such as twitter and Facebook. Great examples of this are the recent twitter chats about the outbreak of Ebola in Western Africa. The CDC tweeted the most updated information and told providers here in the US how to be prepared. This would have been much more difficult in previous years. Now, we have it all available in one place with not much effort to find it. Also, research studies can be spread through social media. Groundbreaking studies and changes in treatment guidelines can be spread to those who need to know in a much more efficient way than hoping physicians happen on the information. Announcements for webinars and other educational events can be announced through social media, drawing in more attendees and making it a much more rewarding educational experience.

4. Building connections: The days of handing out business cards are over. We are no longer only connected to our colleagues and others at the hospital we work at. We can now connect with doctors and others all across the globe. This is made possible in many different platforms: twitter, LinkedIn, Facebook. They all have their own intricacies of how connections are made possible. But, this increased connectivity has the potential to change healthcare around the world. We can share medical information with doctors in other countries. We can learn treatment nuances from those same doctors that we may not have known otherwise. Social media is truly transforming the way healthcare communications are happening. Many doctors are slow to pick up on this very valuable tool and soon will be lost in the system unless they join this modern intercommunication landscape, a landscape that is flourishing before our very eyes. Recently, I was asked for personal advice on

using Twitter. There are many articles out there that say we (physicians) don't know how to properly use social media. Social media can be a very powerful tool in medicine. It can not only help us get medical information out there to our patients, but it can also help us connect with people, colleagues, and organizations to give us more visibility—whether for career advancement, media contacts, or just to get our voices heard.

These are some of the tips I have come up with for doctors who want to take advantage of the many opportunities social media can offer:

1. Never communicate to patients through social media outlets. It is a set up for disaster and HIPAA violations.

2. Social media can be used for educating patients. Patients can follow you on these pages to get information about your practice and whatever medical information you wish to share.

3. Twitter is useful for growing your professional connections. It can be leveraged so you get known and also connect with other doctors, healthcare information technology people, media, etc. Patients can follow you on Twitter, but it generally is not a useful method of providing patient information because tweets are limited to 140 characters.

4. Choose your followers carefully. Block those who spam or troll you ("trolls" are people who negatively post with the deliberate intent of provoking a reaction). Many people will try to sell you things. Monitor your account because it is not uncommon for it to

be hacked.

5. Grow your network. Have a group that you regularly tweet your important messages to so they can share and spread it around, or "retweet" it.

6. Watch your words. It is OK to send out personal tweets sometimes. I find this helpful because it encourages more people to interact with me. I find Twitter feeds that are all business rather boring. People will be more interested if you mix it up.

7. Don't lose your temper. Many people are watching you. If trolled, answer calmly or ignore. Many trolls have groups that will attack if they feel they are being attacked. I am currently being trolled by the anti-vaxxer community because of my advocacy of pro-vaccination. I ignore them. If they send you tweets, no one else sees them unless they put a character in front of your username.

8. Retweet good articles from trusted sources, like the WHO, CDC, or other credible organizations. People will come to see you as a trusted expert and resource.

9. Don't be shy. Social media is meant to be social. Post favorite

tweets, thank people for retweets (or "RTs"), say good morning to get someone's attention. But don't be a spammer or stalker. If someone doesn't respond, move on. Facebook is a better social media outlet to reach patients.

10. Ask patients to follow or like your practice on Facebook.

11. You can create separate pages on Facebook but just one account. I have my personal Facebook page, but I also have a page for the practice and a personal professional page. .

12. Remember you are in the public now. Don't do anything on Facebook that you wouldn't do in public or that you would want to take back. What is posted on-line, stays online.

13. LinkedIn. LinkedIn is a way to strengthen connections for your career. It is like having an online resume.

14. Try to connect to people you know on LinkedIn. You don't need to accept all invitations to connect with people (I made that mistake and now get many unwanted messages from recruiters).

Inside Our Broken Healthcare System

There are now several communities where physicians can collaborate together outside of public scrutiny. The leading such community is Sermo, which is also my favorite. It is physician-only, and doctors are mostly anonymous, which allows the free flow of communication and collaboration. The advantages are just too many to mention but, in general, doctors are not leveraging these benefits to the maximum potential. It is a vehicle where we can join together and get a unified voice heard. We no longer have to feel isolated.

For years, doctors have been working in a vacuum. And it is for exactly this reason that many of the new mandates are being dumped on our heads without taking into account the opinions of doctors and those of us practicing medicine on the frontlines. However, this isolation is eroding the quality of care that we can provide to our patients. Doctors need to come together and regain our collective voice. It is time for us to retake control of our profession and we need real leaders to step up and show us the way. Unless some action is taken, the quality of healthcare in the US will continue to decline and become less accessible for many.

Furthermore, if this change is not driven by doctors, real reform will

never occur. Mandates and regulations cannot be devised sitting

behind a desk not knowing exactly what goes on in exam rooms

across the country. Those on the frontlines need to make our needs

known and determine what fixes need to be undertaken to provide

high quality patient care. No more trying to get a piece of the

healthcare dollars off of doctors' backs. No more trying to remotely

control the system. The voices of doctors need to amplified so that

we can start to repair the authentic problems in the system.

1- . https://www.afsp.org/preventing-suicide/our-education-and-prevention-programs/programs-for-professionals/physician-and-medical-student-depression-and-suicide/facts-about-physician-depression-and-suicide

Chapter 9: Greed, the Outliers

Inside Our Broken Healthcare System

I always cringe when I see people refer to doctors as greedy. The fact is that most doctors truly care about our patients and do the best to give them the most care. Most of us did not go into deep debt to make money. There are much easier ways to make money than going to 8 years of school following high school graduation followed by 3-5 years of residency depending on the specialty. According to the American Association of Medical Colleges, a nonprofit group of US schools, the median cost to attend private medical colleges was $278,455 and for public medical colleges was $207,868 for graduates finishing in 2013. Clearly, medical school is not a fast, easy road to making money. However, this is not universally true. While the vast majority of doctors are driven by doing the best for our patients, there is a very small group that this does not speak true for. There are indeed some doctors who are driven for profit. And most doctors do not respect these doctors: they give us all a bad name. I recently went to see a specialist for a routine exam. Before the doctor even talked to me, his assistant said she was going to allergy test me because I checked off that I have a history of allergies. I explained to her that I have already

been allergy tested and am in fact am receiving weekly

immunotherapy shots. She kept arguing that all patients who have

a history need to be allergy tested. I finally told her to go explain to

the doctor that I did not to be allergy tested because I already have

been and am doing allergy shots. Reluctantly, she went and asked. I

did not do the tests that day and I truly did not need them. The

specialist I was seeing was not the kind that would treat allergy

patients anyway. This was obviously something that was being done

for profit. It saddens me to see so many people believe that doctors

are driven by greed and making money. Claims are made in the

media that doctors do procedures just for profit, even by our

Commander-in-Chief. I am sure most remember his statement that

doctors make more money performing tonsillectomies than with

conservative treatment. But, for the majority of doctors, nothing

can be further from reality.

Doctors are battling many forces everyday on behalf of our

patients; many that will never be seen or be appreciated. There are the prior authorization and prescription refills that fill our days. And we are always available after hours, whether personally or with a shared coverage group. All this work is uncompensated but we do it for the sake of our patients. We do it because this is what they need to have the best care.

Patients don't know how much we truly care about them. Sometimes we stay awake all night worrying that they will be alright until the morning. They don't see us on Christmas morning as we are watching our own children opening their gifts, which we cast aside to answer their call because their child is vomiting. This is our calling. This is what we are supposed to do. Despite what others may believe, we do care about this other child and want them to be well.   We sometimes can feel the fear that is in a patient's eyes, fear of what terrible disease may be lurking inside. We try to stand up to that fear and calm it down. But, sometimes it breaks us down. Sometimes, medicine fails and there is nothing left to offer. Sometimes, doctors go and cry alone because we take the failure of the medical field as our own. Each patient is unique to us. That is why we balk so much at following set guidelines. Each patient needs to be evaluated for who they are and not how they fit on a clinical pathway. It would be much easier to just follow these care plans. But, we care and our patients deserve our best personalized care.

We feel when our patients die, no matter how old and how sick. We are amazed at their fortitude despite suffering. We learn from their strong spirits. We know their passing is a loss to the world and a tragedy to their loved ones.

There may be some outlier doctors who are driven by greed, but this is a tiny minority. Most doctors truly care. And there are many services we do for free, just because we do care, not because we expect any payment in return. When everyone goes to bed at night, there is always a doctor standing by if they are needed.

There have been increased calls for transparency regarding physicians' earning. In 2014, CMS released the reimbursements made to physicians under the Medicare plan. While it seems that it has revealed some of these outliers, this data is not a true

representation of profits made by physicians. It has been much debated and many people are welcoming the new transparency. I have heard people say that doctors are just too whiny and don't want people to know how much they really make. True, there are outliers abusing the system. These providers should be brought to light. But, wouldn't it make more sense that the HHS department investigates these cases themselves? Personally, the publishing of my Medicare earnings doesn't affect me at all. I do not have a large percentage of Medicare patients in my practice. If anyone wanted to look me up, I am probably towards the bottom of earners. No one can accuse me of being one of those "whiny millionaire doctors" that I have seen posted by many.

However, this information can potentially be harmful. Here is why:

1. The information published only shows the gross receipts of doctors. It is not taking into account overhead costs. For certain procedures and surgeries, overhead costs can be a large percentage of this amount. This data does not represent total profit to the doctor, unless someone were to go and subtract out overhead costs. The public is under the false assumption that these numbers represent profit for providers. This is mis-leading and skewed. For example, in my practice, I administer many vaccines. The cost to buy these vaccines is very costly and I am barely above a break-even point after I am paid. Without that knowledge, people would be under the assumption that I am getting paid more than I am.

2. Doctors in certain specialties and doing surgical procedures are going to have higher incomes. People seeing the published data may not understand this. They may compare all doctors across the board. This, too, will give inaccurate impressions.

3. The discussion of money should not come into the exam room. When I am with a patient, I want to be completely focused on their health. Discussions of how much I get paid would distract me from this task.

4. It may be detrimental to the doctor-patient relationship. If a patient is lead to believe a doctor is only interested in making money, how can they trust that physician? Again, there are doctors who may be guilty of this. But, the majority of us genuinely care about our patients.

5. If there are providers guilty of committing fraud, they are making the rest of us look bad. We want them sanctioned and penalized as much as anyone else. HHS should go after these cases. Not cause the public to make potential false cases from someone who may just be working harder with the Medicare population than the rest of us.

6. Other professions do not have their incomes publicized. Some feel that it is unfair to target doctors specifically like this.

7. My earnings have always been transparent to each individual patient. Every patient receives an EOB (explanation of benefits) after their insurance company has sent me a payment. The EOB shows them exactly what I charged, how much I was paid and how much I was required to write off for every service. This is transparency and has always been there. Nothing is hidden as others allege we are trying to do.

In summary, publishing Medicare incomes for physicians will lead to incorrect assumptions and skewed views of data being generated. There is great danger that doctors who are high earners may be painted in an unfavorable light. It has the potential of eroding the doctor-patient relationship. If HHS wants to publish this data, there should be an effort to rid it of mis-interpretations and false assumptions.

Despite this, the fact is that there are some doctors who have lost their calling and are driven by profit. Unfortunately, these doctors get more attention and stereotype us all. We have all heard stories of doctors convicted for committing insurance fraud. These truly are a very small number. But, what happens in this case is that insurance companies need to invest more to prevent fraud and do audits looking for fraudulent claims. This greatly drives up healthcare costs and casts doctors in a negative light. Doctors who do commit fraud deserve to be prosecuted and punished. They are causing great damage to the healthcare system and harming patients by the fact that they are driving up costs for them. Doctors took an oath to do no harm. As doctors, when we realize one of our colleagues is falling into this greedy category, we should not just ignore this. If they are doing a test or procedure that you suspect is not needed on one of our patients, we should question them about it. Also, we should stop referring to these doctors. They are sabotaging our profession. We need to stand up and show that doctors do truly care about our patients. Greed is an evil in any field but particularly more so in physicians.

While avarice in any profession can cause injury, it is more abhorrent in doctors who are in a healing field. Doctors have a special calling to take care of those in vulnerable positions, whether inflicted by diseases or injury. It is not acceptable for them to be taking advantage of these people. Sure, many people are unhappy with the way insurance companies are run and with our shrinking reimbursements but it is never tolerable to inflict this discontent unto patients. Doctors should be held to a higher standard because we are entrusted with more. And patients need to know that doctors generally care about them and are fighting for them every day.

Chapter 10: Dr. Google and

Misinformed patients

Inside Our Broken Healthcare System

The patient brought me 20 pages of "medical" information she printed off a site on the internet. She was convinced there was something seriously wrong with her. She spent several sleepless nights concerned about this Google diagnosis. This diagnosis was probably the furthest thing from what she actually had. Yet, patients always seem to find the worst ailments when they try to diagnose themselves. And this is understandable because the patients fear the symptoms they are having. I see this every day. I love when my patients advocate for themselves but not when they have the wrong information. This can actually be harmful.

Patients are becoming increasing internet and tech savvy these days. And that is generally a good thing. Patients should be empowered users of the healthcare system and advocates for themselves. Searching information on the internet, however, can lead to many different avenues of knowledge. And patients must be leery of Doctor Google.

I generally love when patients bring me articles or data they learned online. It gives me a good starting point in the discussion. However,

I am finding that many patients are being deceived by knowledge that they Googled. Most of the time, it is of no significance. But, there are times when it can be quite dangerous.

How can Googling medical information be dangerous?

1. People are lead into a false sense of security that there is nothing wrong with them. They have a specific complaint and their search lead them to believe nothing further needs to be done. This delays treatment and diseases can be missed in this fashion. If you have a complaint, speak up and discuss it with your doctor. Share your research but listen when the doctor suggests a test. It is still your right to agree or disagree. But, consider all options and just because a celebrity doctor said something, don't assume it is true.

2. Conversely, patients have a symptom and in their research assume the worst is wrong with them. I have had so many patients convinced that they had cancer based on something they Googled. And there is often no way to reassure them otherwise. Unnecessary tests sometimes are done because of this. Sometimes these tests

have complications. If nothing else, it causes unneeded worry and anxiety.

3. Patients can try remedies that can be dangerous or ineffective. There are many alternative medications out there. Some work and some don't. But there are many being promoted to do things that they are simply not capable of doing. For example, I have recently seen silver nanoparticles being promoted as a cure for Ebola. There is no scientific proof for this and would be frankly negligent to recommend an Ebola patient try this. Yet, these companies are selling these products to gullible people. Instead of getting the medical care they need, they are paying money for something that has no science to support. It is easy to see how that can be dangerous.

4. Patients are avoiding recommended medical care because of things they read online. A big example of this is the anti-vaccine movement. Science has proved again and again that vaccines save lives and are safe. Yet, when some people hear celebrities speaking of the dangers of vaccines, some tend to believe these famous

people and not the test of science. This is exposing people to more deadly infections.

5. Patients are increasingly seeking medical consultations online. While this is a great convenience for many, it is not without dangers. A doctor prescribing antibiotics over the phone can only give a best assumption. Without a hands-on examination, there is simply no way to know exactly what is wrong with you. And how well do you know an online doctor?

While Googling medical information is exposing people to dangers, there is much good available information out there. Patients need to learn as much as they can to be proper advocates in the healthcare system. It behooves everyone to find trusted references to use when information is needed. And online information can never replace a doctor's in person opinion. Your doctor has your best interests at heart.

Telemedicine is all over the media lately. Simply put, it is the use of telecommunications and information technologies to practice medicine remotely. It has been shown to save lives in rural areas where distance is a barrier for patients to be seen in person. It has greatly aided critical care and emergency treatment where time is of the essence. It may involve videoconferences between doctors, sharing radiology studies for others to interpret, or simply giving the patient medical advice over the phone.

While telemedicine has been shown to save lives, should it be the mainstream in medicine? Can it replace office visits as some people are claiming? Should it? Sure, it is very convenient for the patient and cuts overhead costs for the doctors. However, it simply can never replace the face to face doctor patient relationship.

Telemedicine has many useful purposes. It saves lives in remote areas where distance and time are major barriers to transport patients. Additionally, the benefits of having a radiologist review imagining studies are obvious. These studies can be interpreted without the patient present. As wearable technology grows, being able to get access to the information collected becomes more necessary. Being able to watch such data remotely would be a very powerful.

However, traditional medicine should not be replaced by

telemedicine, which is a very powerful tool when used

appropriately. Patients still need real hands on examinations done

by physicians. For example, a cough may have many causes

including pneumonia, bronchitis, asthma, GERD, post-nasal drip,

allergies and many more. There is no way to know just by a given

history over the phone. Auscultation of the lungs and other

examination needs to be done to decide the most probable cause.

Similarly, an earache may not be an ear infection. Any diagnoses

provided by history over the phone or internet are best guesses.

Often, physical examination can eliminate many of these. Many

times patients think they need antibiotics when they do not. To just

prescribe an antibiotic over the phone is contributing to the

epidemic of antibiotic resistance. Unless we limit this prescribing to

only bacterial infections, we soon will have few antibiotics left to

cure these infections.

Telemedicine can also increase bad outcomes because things are

missed when the patient is not seen. Masses in the neck cannot be felt over the phone. Sometimes I see a patient who just looks pale and I know something is wrong. As medical students, we all learned the smell of a Pseudomonas infection. There are just too many things that can be missed or misdiagnosed by remote medicine. It should be truly reserved for those instances where it saves lives and improves care, not for convenience by patients or profit by physicians.

How should telemedicine be used appropriately?

– It has been shown to be invaluable in remote areas. Doctors can get expert help from colleagues which they would not be able to get otherwise because of distance and time constraints.

– Radiologists can read imaging studies remotely, making diagnoses more quickly at times when they may have not otherwise been available.

– Remote data collection for various disease states can aid in controlling certain medical conditions. Patients with pacemakers have been doing this for years. Technology is available to be able to check the function of pacemakers and send this data over the phone. We should expect to see a proliferation of this type of technology.

– For established patients who doctors know well and are comfortable knowing their medical condition. It should never be used to diagnose new disease, like diabetes or hypertension. While telemedicine has very great potential to change the way medicine is practiced, caution needs to be exercised. With all the press about telemedicine, patients feel their doctors should always be available. And I am, by telephone. The other day, I was driving to work and a patient called. When I answer my cell, I say my name but I guess the patient didn't hear or just didn't expect the doctor to pick up the office phone line. She was trying to schedule an appointment. I gave her my hours and the patient said, "That is ridiculous, she should be there in the evening. Those hours don't work for me".   There was another doctor there in the evening but she wanted only me. And I work 3 evenings a week. Information out there sets the expectation that doctors need to treat patients at all hours of the day. This simply is undoable. We are human too. The burnout rate among physicians is higher than it has ever been. And

this demands being placed on us is making it even harder.

Telemedicine can be a great tool. However, it is often being utilized

in the wrong way. Patients are looking for the easy way, they want

to avoid an office visit. Many call looking for a prescription for

antibiotics. And many of them get what they want. But, this is

leading to a very dangerous disaster in our country: antibiotic

resistance. We are seeing this on a more frequent basis. Antibiotics

that used to work for certain infections no longer work. And some

of these infections now require 2 or even 3 antibiotics to cure. No

new antibiotics have been developed in recent years. And the ones

we have are becoming useless. We need to prescribe these

medications judiciously. And we need to use telemedicine in an

appropriate way.

Many patients fall under the spell of **pseudoscience**, those things

that have no real scientific evidence supporting that they work or

are safe. I recently had a supporter of nano-silver particles tweet

me a study that it cures Ebola. But, after reading it carefully, it was just a well devised promotional piece. And it would kill people to use it as a cure for Ebola, a disease which has no cure at the present moment. It is easy to see how evidence lacking studies can be harmful. Another current hot item is essential oils. They are purported to cure all ills, from dementia to depression to bowel problems. Yet, there is no evidence that they work. These products fall outside the jurisdiction of the FDA. So, there are really no safety standards. They could put anything in them and there is no one to test it to see if it is safe. And they are very costly. So, if you pay out big dollars, you are buying something that has no proof that it works and no proof that it is safe. Yet, many people believe in their healing powers based on what they read on the internet. Often, these products are endorsed by celebrities. If they use them, they must be safe, right? Not really. They are just being paid to attach their name to these products.

How can you tell if something is effective and safe?

-The studies being quoted have been done on a large number of patients, particularly in the thousands. Most of the pseudoscience ones have subject numbers in the 10's.

- The site or information is supported by a large well-known organization, such as the CDC or WHO.

- It can stand scrutiny of healthcare professionals. Take it to your doctor and ask. Ask any nurses you know. You will begin to see the consensus of the medical field.

- If it sounds kooky, it probably is.

- If someone is selling a product, they are probably just looking for business. They may publish misleading information to achieve that goal.

- It should be FDA approved. Anything that has not withstood testing by the FDA has not been proven safe. Furthermore, the ingredients are not even verified.

Another area where patients can get misleading and harmful information is from the anti-vaxxer community. In California, there has been a recent outbreak of Pertussis (whooping cough) and a 1 year old died from it. This is a disease that is preventable by a vaccine. Yet, there is much "pseudoscience" being spread about the dangers of vaccines. They quote articles, which upon scrutiny, fail to stand up to science. Yet, many people are easily duped by them. Because of the movement of avoiding vaccines, we are seeing a rise in the number of cases of Pertussis, Measles, and Mumps over the past few years. These diseases were nearly eradicated by the immunization initiative set forth by the CDC

 I don't blame patients for being demanding; they are being crushed by the broken system. They are trying to be made well and stay safe in a system that has deserted their best interests. They are asked to pay more and more for less and less. And they receive so much conflicting information, not only in regards to medicine but insurance coverage as well. And large amounts of money are being spent on their data while at the same time they are being denied needed medical services. I think anyone can see the wrong in this

situation. It is time to care about the patient again. And welcome

their advocacy for their own healthcare. Doctors need to step up

and help patients find medical information that is truly sound and

meaningful for patients.

Chapter 11: The Push for Big Data

Big data seems to be a key point that many are pushing these days.
It seems many have lost sight of the person in the patient and care
more about the data surrounding them. Insurance companies and
the government are devising ways of gathering this data
surrounding the patients. The healthcare and technology industries
are being inundated with information about implementing big data.
Software vendors are making systems that will eventually be able to
talk to each other so that a patient's data will be readily available
from just about anywhere and to just about anywhere. While that
reality is still out of reach, do we really want that much data? An
argument can be made that the government and insurance
companies need to track these metrics to evaluate patient
outcomes and physician performances. But, are these large
quantities of data truly helpful or necessary for providing the best
medical care to patients? From my own expert experience as a
practicing physician, I would have to answer no. So many metrics
are now charted in the medical record that it becomes difficult to

abstract what is truly necessary for treating the patient in front of me. To qualify for meaningful use, certain metrics need to be charted; which are often variables not relevant to the current patient's visit. But, if they are not charted, I will not be using my EMR meaningfully according to government regulations. While presently that would disqualify me for EMR incentive bonuses, in the future, that would cost me financially in the terms of penalties for failing to meaningfully adapt an EMR system. Many of my patients are seen by doctors in other specialties. We are often requesting these records. It becomes a search and rescue mission to find what medications have been prescribed by other providers. While this can be quite time consuming and frustrating, there are often times a delay can pose a danger. I had a pediatric patient come with difficulty breathing. The patient was recently seen by a cardiologist. I did have those records faxed over but it took time to search out the cardiac testing that had been done on the patient. If the symptoms had been the result of a cardiac disease, this search through the maze of records would have cost valuable time in starting appropriate treatment in this child. While EMRs have great potential to make our charts more legible and efficient, we need to tailor the data to what is truly relevant to patient care. Now, it is becoming near outlawed to copy and paste patient notes in their medical record. I personally free hand all my notes. But, if we are required, as an example, to document smoking status at every single visit and the patient continues smoking 1 pack per day, how many different ways are there seriously to chart that? Sure there are lazy doctors who copy and paste and the EMR suffers for lack of accuracy. But, these are the outliers. The great majority of physicians truly care about documentation. We realize it is not just a medical record but a legal document. And it can truly be used against us.

I think the time has come to stop the supersizing of big data in medical records. It is slowing doctors down and causing inefficiencies in the system, which can occasionally have dangerous outcomes. Let data be what it needs to be: useful information that drives medicine and treatment of the patient. Perhaps the opportunity has arrived to downsize the medical chart to the data

that is clinically meaningful to the ones that need to use them for

patient care.

Why is there such a big push for big data?

- Insurance companies are using this data to track clinical

  outcomes. They use this data to track specific diseases, such

  as diabetes or hypertension, and then target a specific

  outcome to track, such as HbA1C or cholesterol level. While

  improving these measures is a great ideal, this is not how

  the data is being used. Rather, it is being used to evaluate

  the quality of a given doctor. Many doctors are angered by

  this because many of these variables are subject to the

  control of the patient. For example, if I have a patient who

  eats McDonald's every day, I will never be able to get their

  cholesterol under control no matter what measures I

  employ. Yet, insurance companies are proposing financial

  penalties for doctors who don't meet insurance company

specified outcomes. This is not just harmful to doctors but patients as well. What will likely happen is that some doctors will stop treating high risk and non-compliant patients. These patients will likely have worse outcomes trying to find access to medical care and will drive up healthcare costs.

- The FDA is using big data analytics to analyze drug safety. While this may seem to be a good thing, some question the way it is being done. Most of the data is gathered from doctors' billing information rather than the patients' medical charts. They may be searching patients on a particular drug and then will look at the billing data to see if the prescribing doctor submitted any billing code for such things as intestinal problems for a given period afterwards. Anyone can see how this would be prone to error as there is no way to make an exact correlation without the actual medical record.

- Data can be used to compare physicians' practicing habits. We often get analyses that show how our ER visits, prescribing habits, or ordering of certain tests or medications compare to other doctors in the same specialty. While this can be a good tool as well to spot outliers, it is not as simple as it is proposed. Some doctors work with higher risk populations. Some limit their practices to certain ages and certain diseases. Yet, these variables are not calculated into these analyses. So true comparisons are not being made without these confounding elements being taken into account. Insurance companies are trying to make these comparisons.

- Data is also being abstracted about doctors' billing information. Some of this is to detect fraud. But, many doctors feel that it is more so the insurance companies can search for anyway to get out of paying claims. We are seeing more and more denied or delayed payments for clean claims.

We frequently get insurance company representatives come to review charts. Most of the time, they do not know how to use our EHR and want to print out pages and pages of records. We have to have a staff sit down and explain our system to them. There are so many systems now available. It makes the task almost impossible. While data and data analytics can be a valuable tool in healthcare, it needs to be used in the right way. It is very important that all this data is protected and not prone to being leaked. Patients need to be assured that their HIPAA rights will not be violated. Data should be used for improving clinical outcomes and establishing medication safety. It still has a ways to go in this regards. It should not be a tool for penalizing doctors for not being good data entry clerks and reporting requested metrics. This is exactly what is happening under the CQHA program. Many doctors are now being docked 1% of their reimbursements from Medicare for not submitting the required information. For this to be successful there needs to be a team effort between these agencies and doctors. As

it exists, these mandates are decided largely by non-

physicians and then mandated onto physicians to comply.

We will never get anywhere with this model. Doctors need

to step up to take the lead and other need to hear doctors'

voices. It is not acceptable to demand big data out of

doctors without knowing how it is affecting our care of our

patients.

Chapter 12: Drug Abuse and

Prescription Medications

I see many patients who come in requesting prescriptions for Percocet or some other controlled substance when obviously they don't need. Every doctor can tell many stories of made up tales in this regards. We hear how these medications "fell in the toilet" or were "eaten by the dog". This rarely happens with medications that are not controlled substances. Most doctors are able to detect red flags of apparently drug-seeking patients. Patients can

make up wild stories in order to obtain a prescription for a controlled medication. I have had a woman tell me she has Hodgkin's Lymphoma and she was in severe pain. She knew most doctors would be sympathetic to her diagnosis. However, upon obtaining and reviewing her records, she was obviously making up this medical history. Another patient left behind his wallet. He had been arguing strenuously for a Percocet prescription. When we looked in his wallet to see who it belonged to, he had picture IDs with 5 different names, none of which was the one he gave to us.

Inside Our Broken Healthcare System

Why do patients go to such extremes to get these medications? One reason is that they are highly habit-forming. Many people are simply addicted to them and need them. After they have been taking them for some time, tolerance sets in and they need higher and higher doses to get the same effect. Hence, they need to find more sources and start to "doctor shop". In many states now, there is a database for controlled substances. I can look up any prescription that was filled for a given patient for these medications. I once had a woman asking for Percocet and when I searched her in the database, she had 23 pages of prescriptions filled in the last 6 months from 5 different doctors and 3 different pharmacies. These databases are a great tool. However, they are limited in that they are not yet available in every state. And I cannot search prescriptions that were filled in other states. Some patients use different names to fill medications and there is no way to know this.

Another reason for this controlled substance epidemic is that it is a very profitable business. Many people make much money off diverting these medications. I have been told that in my area, 1 tablet of Percocet sells on the street for $20. So, if a patient has a prescription for 30 tablets, he can make $600 from selling them. And, in most cases, his insurance covers the cost of filling this medication so he/she is not paying anything out of pocket. Now, if that same patient goes to 5 or 6 different doctors, you can easily see how profitable it can become. Drug diversion of these medications has become a huge problem in the US.

I have reported a few patients to the police who I suspected were diverting medications. However, the narcotics agents are so over-whelmed, they simply do not have time to pursue all these cases. They are looking for the big cases where they can arrest the biggest number of people. They want to break these drug chains. Often, these patients are not working with others and it is just not worth going after these individuals. And the law is not very punitive in these cases. The biggest issue with the diversion of drugs is that it often targets kids in schools. Prescription drug addiction is harmful in and of itself. However, there are now many studies suggesting that it is the gateway drug to bigger addictions, namely IV heroin

use. Prescription drugs have been relatively easy to obtain. Some

kids just get it out of grandma's medicine cabinet. The problem is

that in recent years there has been a much bigger crackdown on

prescribing these medications. So, a person that had a relatively

easy time obtaining the medication that they are addicted to now

finds it more and more difficult to obtain and it has gotten more

costly. The alternative that is available that will give them the same

high is IV heroin. In many cases it is now cheaper to obtain. And this

is much more addictive. The incidence in IV heroin is seeing a surge

in many communities across the US. And it is particularly hitting

teens. Much potential of our youth is being lost to this epidemic.

And I have seen several patients in my practice who desperately

want help. But, that help is not so easy to find. Many insurance

companies do not cover these rehab services. And there are long

waits to get into these programs.

Why is prescription drug abuse harmful to our healthcare system?

-It drives up costs by directly paying for medications that are not indicated. This is healthcare dollars lost for no good reason. In the age where we are all now trying to be more cost conscious, this contradicts all these efforts that we are doing.

-It drives up costs by the harm that it causes. People have adverse medical outcomes from the use of these agents. People frequently overdose leading to expensive hospital stays. Rehab programs are costly.

-It is damaging lives and making people unemployable. More people are living off the state. Their addiction prevents them from being gainfully employed.

- It is harming our nation's youth. Many are falling victim to this epidemic.

- It prevents patients who need these medications from being able to obtain them. Many doctors now get their suspicions aroused just by the mention of the names of these medications. But there are patients who truly need them to control the pain.

They are made to feel like drug seekers when they are merely trying to get medical treatment for their ailments. These patients are being very much hurt by this epidemic.

Over the past few years, prescription drug abuse has blossomed. Some recent control has been seen leading to an increase in IV heroin use. We truly need to curb the abuse of these agents and prescribe them only when truly indicated. It is not just increasing costs to our healthcare system, but it is destroying lives. Doctors need to lead in this fight. Many patients play on the doctors' sympathies. As a doctor, it is hard to see a patient who is in pain and not want to help them. We need to learn the red flags of when patients are playing us. We need to search those databases and ask for records. Unless the abuse of these medications is halted, we are facing another very real crisis. And this one has the potential to damage very many lives.

damage very many lives.

Conclusion

Who Broke the System?

Inside Our Broken Healthcare System

Clearly, the American healthcare system is broken and harming healthcare professionals and patients alike. Patients are not getting the care they deserve, whether it is due to be uninsured or having inadequate coverage or it is because the system is dysfunctional. Doctors and other healthcare professionals are bearing the brunt of the impact that healthcare changes are heralding. And most often, we are in disagreement with many of these changes. Patients are increasingly frustrated with finding a doctor, getting tests and medications they need, and paying for out-of-pocket expenses. Numerous doctors are disenchanted with their career choice and burnout is a common complaint. Frequently, doctors are now looking to retire early or for alternate career paths. Treating patients has become unfulfilling for many due to administrative burdens, increasing government regulations, and overbearing insurance over-sight. Doctors fight daily to get procedures and medications covered that their patients need. Most often, the battle is with someone who is not even a doctor or has any clue about the patient. These daily battles become wearing.

Additionally, doctors now have to fight on a more abundant basis to get paid for services they provided. Their incomes are stagnant or shrinking while overhead costs are soaring. Increasingly, doctors are selling out their practices and joining large groups and hospitals. How can any of these changes have a positive impact on the system when those on the frontlines are not buying into it?

So, who broke it?

Many people look to put blame on doctors for the broken healthcare system. Yet, it has been years since doctors truly had any control over it. More often these days, doctors are treated like pawns and servants, our independence and integrity being worn away and questioned. But, who really is to blame for the broken healthcare system?

1. Commercial insurance companies who have no oversight and profit from denying services to patients. I have seen more and more diagnostic tests and medications being denied since I started practicing approximately 15 years ago. All too commonly, procedures and medications require prior-authorizations. This is time-consuming and costly. Insurance companies employ people just for this task. Some get bonuses for cost containment. The executives of these insurance companies make obscene salaries. Meanwhile, they are tying doctors hands from doing what is needed to provide patients with the best quality medical care. Medicine is now driven for cost-containment rather than quality

thanks to the for-profit insurance companies.

2. The government has been placing increasing burdens on regulating physicians. One good example of this is the Meaningful Use EHR program. While we are now able to get a bonus for qualifying for implementing an EHR system, soon doctors will be penalized for not complying. The process to get qualified is onerous and truly not meaningful for doctors. Doctors spend time checking boxes to record metrics so that we don't get penalized. We rather use that time to devote to our patients.

3. The tort system has also had a disastrous effect on the healthcare system. While patients should have the means to be compensated for obvious negligence and malpractice, this is not what is occurring. Frivolous lawsuits make up a great majority of cases. Patients often threaten the doctor with lawsuits if we do not give into their demands. Doctors pay large premiums on their malpractice insurance for just this reason. For some specialties, such as obstetrics, it has become too expensive a premium to continue in their specialty. Much medicine is driven by the need to

avoid getting sued. Not only does this drive up costs, but it erodes the trust between doctors and patients. There is a big need for tort reform.

4. Groups like the AMA who pander to politicians more than anyone else. When they say they speak up for doctors, the public listens. However, many doctors feel that their voice is not our voice. They are not listening to doctor's concerns about what is needed to improve healthcare in this country.

While the healthcare system pushes forward in need of repair, doctors continue at what they do best: treating patients. Few people became doctors for the income. Many claim that doctors are driven by profit yet this is not true in most cases. The vast majority of doctors care about our patients and want to offer the highest care for our patients.

Instead of handing down more mandates in a lame attempt to improve healthcare, perhaps the time has come to ask those on the frontlines for their input on how to fix this broken system. The doctors' voices need to be heard. We see all the damage that is being caused by the broken system. Unless, regulators know this, there is absolutely no way that they can devise any mandates to fix it. And the doctors practicing clinical medicine rather than the academic physicians and their theories should be listened to. Doctors need to step up and take the lead.

The healthcare system in the US leads the world in new technologies and medical break-throughs being discovered and created. But, what good is it having the best medicine in the world when patients cannot afford to utilize it?

The patient has become lost in our new world of medicine. Battles are being played out behind the scenes to see how to profit from them. The same is happening to doctors. The time has come to put the patient back at center stage where they belong. We need to focus on their humanity more than their metrics. We need to stand up to the forces that are dehumanizing them. Rather than fighting useless mandates, we should be fighting for the lives and health of our patients. Doctors need to take back our profession.

There simply is no one else who cares enough about patients to do it. And patients need to take a stand against the entities that are denying them access to quality of care. It is time for the doctor and patient to become a team again. The time has come to repair this broken system.

When I go into the exam room and close the door, I face my patient and am again reminded of why I became a doctor: to alleviate suffering. And no matter how broken the system becomes, that person in front of me is truly the most important thing that matters and I will continue my daily fight to get the best for them.

Who wants to help?